Praise for

Reversing Your Child's Eating Disorder

"This account of one family's journey into and out of the maelstrom of anorexia nervosa is stirring, insightful, and informative. Parents of children with eating disorders will find this book helpful, supportive, and deeply moving."

– James Lock. MD, PhD, Department of Psychiatry,
Stanford University School of Medicine;
Director of the Adolescent Eating Disorders Program,
author of *Help Your Teenager with Their Eating Disorder*

"Boys and men get eating disorders and can die from them the same way as girls and women. In this intensely honest story of illness and recovery, we are taken on a journey from the edge of death to a healthy life. The critical understanding of the biology of eating disorders, the need for family based therapy and parental leadership in weight restoration, the role of validation and love for the sufferer are all beautifully explained and referenced. As a treatment professional and a man in recovery from Anorexia Nervosa, I highly recommend this very important book."

– Mark Warren, MD, MPH Chief Medical Officer,
The Emily Program, Cleveland Center for Eating Disorders

"There is such power in hearing from another parent that there is hope and that the parental role is not only important but essential to the process of recovery. This book cries out for better treatment, better science, and for fully engaged parents."

– Laura Collins, author of *Eating With Your Anorexic* and *Throwing Starfish Across the Sea*

"When parents are faced with the overwhelming reality that their child has a life-threatening illness like Anorexia Nervosa, it is invaluable to know that other parents have faced and survived similar challenges. The author details the path she and her son took to help him fully recover, which will surely serve as a helpful guide to families that find themselves caught in the confusing frenzy of a new diagnosis."

~ Rhonda Lee Benner, LCSW, Licensed Clinical Social Worker and Certified Family-Based Treatment Therapist The New England Eating Disorders Program at Mercy Hospital

"A passionate portrayal of a mother's desperate journey to understand her precious son's descent into anorexia. This journal is an amazing 'how to' that loved ones of those afflicted will cling to and one in which they will recover hope. I am grateful for her faith which guided her through this nightmare and led her to help her son when he was unable to do so himself. A must read!"

~ Judith Walker, MEd, DCH, LPCC, Master of Education, Doctor of Clinical Hypnotherapy, Licensed Professional Clinical Counselor

"This memoir reveals that by *embracing* the unpredictable events of a destructive disorder, you are able to experience healing and a sense of purpose in the midst of pain and confusion. These pages tell a real heartfelt life story of hope enlivened by faith *and*, truly, a new lease on life."

~ Dr. Clement Marcantonio, LMFT, Licensed Marriage and Family Therapist, Professor of Counseling Psychology

"Every parent who worries about his or her child's eating behaviors needs to read this story and be armed with preventative and responsive action."

~ Kellie Lavender, Registered Psychotherapist and Certified Family-Based Treatment Therapist, New Zealand

"This book offers a unique parental/clinician perspective on implementing a life-saving treatment that research has shown to be crucial in effectively treating Anorexia Nervosa and other Eating Disorders."

~ Maria-Christina Stewart, Ph.D.

"Accessing seemingly insurmountable odds, Jessica shares life lessons in hurdling emotional, mental, financial, and relationship obstacles to help her son recover from anorexia. This is an inspiring story for every parent that teaches strength in the face of challenge."

~ Shari Au, Ph.D., LLC, Psychologist

"This book is a must read, not only for parents of children with eating disorders, but also for clinicians. Jessica merges her clinical training and maternal instincts to provide a practical guide for anyone interested in learning more about caring for someone with an eating disorder. I highly recommend this book!"

~ Melissa N. Green, Psy.D.,
Licensed Clinical Psychologist

"*Reversing Your Child's Eating Disorder* is a poignant memoir of a dedicated mother and clinician fighting tirelessly for her child's health on an indelible journey. Reading about her unwavering spirit in this detailed account of healing will provide hope to any parent struggling with this dangerous and deadly disease."

~ Jessica Motroni, LMFT,
Licensed Marriage and Family Therapist

"A genuine, honest and informative account of one family's courage to go head-to-head with this disorder. The book offers great insight into the reality of the situation and the depth of emotional turmoil a mother experiences when faced with helping her son battle against anorexia nervosa. *Reversing Your Child's Eating Disorder* is a great supportive reference offering a sense of mirroring and a pathway to express the emotion-laden material that many families struggling with an eating disorder often experience."

~ Monique Hess, MA, LMFT, Master of Arts,
Licensed Marriage and Family Therapist

"A compelling and heartfelt account of the powerful influence eating disorders have on individuals and the people close to them. This book is a must-read for anyone impacted by eating disorders personally or through their professional work."

~ Lisa Heiden-Kimball, LMHC,
Licensed Mental Health Counselor

"Until I read *Healing a Hijacked Mind*, I truly had no idea how devastating anorexia can be, and for a parent, it is all the more terrifying. Jessica Goering shows a mother's true love and heroism in getting to the bottom of what caused her son's eating disorder and finding ways to rebuild her family's life. Anyone facing a similar situation will find strength, hope, and a path to action in these pages."

— Tyler R. Tichelaar, Ph.D., Award-Winning Author of
The Best Place and Narrow Lives

"*Healing a Hijacked Mind* is the story of an unexpected and unsolicited journey. One that depicts a mother's horror facing the near loss of her son who was suddenly stricken with anorexia nervosa, terrorized by fear, and filled with pain and grief. But more than that, it is a story of the healing power of love. And the courage and unyielding faith that brought together a family and a community to heal a child."

~ Loren Breithoff, LMFT-AT, Licensed Marriage
and Family Therapist—Art Therapist

"Parents of children with any life-threatening issue will find this book truly informative. This book should be on every Parent Education shelf in libraries, schools, and therapists' offices."

~ Barbara Gosselin, MS, LMFT, Master of Science,
Licensed Marriage and Family Therapist, Educator

"Once you start reading, you won't be able to put this book down. Jessica's emotional personal journey witnessing her child's malnourished condition and finding ways to help him heal and regain his health are enthralling and inspiring."

~ Emmy Agustin, MS, CCLS, Master of Science,
Certified Child Life Specialist

"This book is a must read for every parent to insure that you will spot the early signs of anorexia and treat it before it is too late."

~ Patrick Snow, International Best-Selling Author of
Creating Your Own Destiny and *Boy Entrepreneur*

"This shocking memoir by Jessica Goering opens a portal into the anorexic mind and a window into the home of a mother willing to do whatever it takes to reclaim the life of her son. Jessica shares practical tips for desperate parents on how to take action and help their child battle this life-threatening illness."

~ Jeff Bow, Author of *Stop Thinking, Start Believing*

"HOPE. One word to describe the emotion elicited by reading *Reversing Your Child's Eating Disorder: Healing a Hijacked Mind to Overcome Anorexia*. Parents be empowered!"

~ Joe Lopez, Author of *Creating the Champion Within*

"Jessica Goering's book, *Reversing Your Child's Eating Disorder: Healing a Hijacked Mind to Overcome Anorexia*, forever changed my level of empathy for sufferers of eating disorders as well as their shell-shocked families. The heart and soul behind this story is evident, and this gripping memoir will help others traverse their own path to healing."

~ Lori Chaffin, Author of *Messages Straight from the Heart*

"From start to finish this book will pull on your heartstrings. The most traumatic event a human being can experience is the loss of a child. As you turn the pages, you can feel the palpable pain of a mother in distress as she desperately tries to stop this trauma as it threatens to become her reality. You won't be able to put the book down!"

~ Mele Huddy, Author of *Leading with Your Dreams*

REVERSING YOUR CHILD'S EATING DISORDER

HEALING A HIJACKED MIND TO OVERCOME ANOREXIA

JESSICA GOERING, LMHC, NCC

AVIVA PUBLISHING
New York

Reversing Your Child's Eating Disorder
Healing a Hijacked Mind to Overcome Anorexia

Published by:
Aviva Publishing
Lake Placid, NY
(518) 523-1320
www.avivapubs.com

Address all inquiries to:
Jessica Goering
(808) 798-9979
Email: Jessica@ReversingYourChildsEatingDisorder.com

www.ReversingYourChildsEatingDisorder.com
www.JessicaGoering.com

ISBN: 978-1-940984-44-5
Library of Congress: 2014945847

Editor: Tyler Tichelaar
Cover Design: Nicole Gabriel /Angel Dog Productions
Interior Book Design: Nicole Gabriel /Angel Dog Productions

Printed in the United States of America

First Edition

2 4 6 8 10 12

The thing that is really hard,
and really amazing,
is giving up on being perfect and
beginning the work of being yourself.

— Anna Quindlen

DEDICATION

To my boys:

Thank you for being YOU. Period. I cannot imagine not getting to be your mom and all that entails. There is no secret (I tell everyone!) that motherhood is my favorite job. And not just a job—a privilege, an opportunity, a calling, and a blessing without description. My one prayer is that you honor God with your lives and realize that your specific qualities, attributes, and capabilities are replicated from the image of the Almighty and are designed to show His love to this world. You are a conduit of that love. The vessel is exactly as it should be. Know, truly know, your inherent value and Who determines that value and has said, "It is good."

To my readers:

Thank you for picking up this book and opening up your mind to the story these pages hold. My hope is that you gain knowledge and awareness about eating disorders from our journey, and at minimum, you will increase your empathy for those who suffer from this terrible illness. But beyond that, hopefully you will become a helping hand to those who need their lives, health, and futures back.

ACKNOWLEDGMENTS

I sincerely wish to recognize and thank those who came alongside my sons and me during this battle for health and sanity. They provided emotional support, practical assistance, childcare, medical advice, written words of hope, spiritual guidance, and prayer.

Ingrid Middleton, Heath and Kirsten Hollenbeck, Taylor Graham, Pastor Matt and Cyndi Dirks and the entire Harbor Church Ohana, the staff at UnNamed Middle School with special thanks to Angie Inouye and Wayne Matsukawa, Dr. Laurie Edwards, Ph.D., the staff at Rogers Memorial Hospital with special thanks to Dr. Erik Ulland, the Adolescent Medicine staff at Tripler Army Medical Center with special thanks to Colonel Jeffrey Greene, MD, Andrew Warren Osten, MD., and Sean Carroll, MD, the staff at 15th Group Medical Hickam Air Force Base with special thanks to Captain Caroline Williams, MD, Captain Shaina Rogers, MD, and Amelia Walker, Dr. Pia Francisco-Natanauan, Josiah and Hannah Goering, James and Gloria Goering, Andrew and Victoria Jergenson, Rik and Sue Reuter, Michael and Angela Fitzpatrick, Mary Ann Crawford, Loren Breithoff, Shari Au, James Lock, MD., Ph.D., Dr. Daniel Le Grange, Laura Collins, and the Eating Disorder Association of America.

I also thank those whose efforts and support enabled this book to reach completion:

Patrick Snow, Nicole Gabriel, MBA, Susan Friedmann, James Lock,

MD., Ph.D., Lisa Heiden-Kimball, LMHC, Judith Walker, MEd, DCH, LPCC, Jessica Motroni, LMFT, Monique Hess, MA, LMFT, Shari Au, Ph.D., LLC., Dr. Clement Marcantonio, Melissa N. Green, PsyD., Loren Breithoff LMFT-AT., Barbara Gosselin MS, LMFT., Emmy Agustin, MS, CCLS, Joe Lopez, Mele Huddy, Lori Chaffin, Jeff Bow, Laura Collins, Rhonda Lee Benner, LCSW, Kellie Lavender, Maria-Christina Stewart, Ph.D, and Mark Warren, MD, MPH.

With a special note of thanks to my talented editor, Tyler Tichelaar, for his superb understanding of language, skillful adherence to all things grammar, and dedication to ensuring this book most effectively conveyed the message intended by this author.

CONTENTS

People need to be helped.
People still think eating disorders are a choice;
they are not.

— Cindy Jackson

FOREWORD

Eating disorders kill. Statistically speaking, anorexia and bulimia have the highest morbidity rates of any psychiatric illness.

Once an eating disorder enters a person's life, it becomes the mask and the mirror, hiding the truth from self and reflecting back an image that encompasses every painful feeling and every frightening thought, into one word: FAT.

That word still scares me, even after all these years. I have suffered and recovered and suffered from anorexia and bulimia since the age of fourteen. The same age of the precious boy this book is so soulfully written about by his mother.

Treatment for eating disorders was formerly punitive and limited. My own downward spiral to fifty-nine pounds took me far from my family and into a world of tubes and scales, as well as unruly helpers who really knew nothing about treating a starving teenager, except by re-feeding. This re-feeding process is still, to this day, one of the most traumatic incidents of my memory—being made to feel alone and like a bad person because I was having a hard time gaining weight. My thinness was my identity, and they were taking it away from me!

I entered the world of Jessica and her son through a short but terrifying phone call.

Her son had stopped eating, had become sullen, and was a stark shadow of his formerly beautiful, vibrant self.

Having just moved to Hawaii, Jessica contended with issues and stresses in terms of finding the right help, and since her son was on the mainland with his father, Jessica felt desperate to do something. As I listened to her, I found myself wishing my own mother had an opportunity to connect with resources that might have made my illness less lengthy and less life-consuming, but my immediate response was finding first inpatient care to arrest the current starvation, then follow up care closely guarded by professionals as soon as he was able to return to Hawaii.

That return marked the beginning of a healing journey that Jessica and her sons embarked upon, unaware of the subsequent challenges that would arise. With each phone call, email, and text, I watched and listened as this dedicated mother stood by her son, pushing through the behaviors, toward the center, where the truth and love lie and remain.

It is that struggle that is so eloquently detailed in this book—one that Jessica has written to detail her experience as mother, as professional, as healer, and as a person of great love and faith. Her healthy son is a testament to her steadfast efforts and proof that families can heal and take back control of the destructive eating disorders that can only disappear with diligent, vigilant focus and a great deal of love.

Ingrid Middleton LCSW, MSW, MS,
Licensed Clinical Social Worker,
Master of Social Work, Master of Science
Author of *The Secret of Healing By Touch*

Deception is the word I most associate with anorexia
and the treachery which comes from falsehood.
The illness appears inviting.
It would seem to offer something to those unwary or
unlucky enough to suffer from it – friendship,
a get-out, or a haven - when, in fact, it is a trap.

— Carol Lee

INTRODUCTION:

THE LIFE STEALER

Anorexia Nervosa is the most deadly psychiatric disorder known to man. If you are going to roll the mental illness dice, you don't want to land on *AN*. This illness can be a death sentence—a slow, tortuous, painful one. According to the American Psychological Association, "People with anorexia nervosa have a distorted body image that causes them to see themselves as overweight even when they're dangerously thin. Often refusing to eat, exercising compulsively, and developing unusual habits such as refusing to eat in front of others, they lose large amounts of weight and may even starve to death." (1) This disorder causes more fatalities than any other diagnosis in the mental health field. And when you reference the *Diagnostic and Statistical Manual of Mental Disorders, Fifth Edition*, the *DSM-5*, more than 300 terms exist to describe a range of human experiences gone awry. Yet, anorexia nervosa ranks first for stealing life breath from its sufferer. In fact, the National Institute of Mental Health (NIMH) estimates the death rate to be around 10 percent. (2)

Hold up ten fingers and think of ten people in your life who struggle with eating in any realm. Now imagine their struggle is with self-induced starvation. Then take one away and the finger stump represents the loss of one of those precious souls. That number is too high to ignore. This illness robs parents of their children and children of their parents. NIMH further estimates that this life stealer afflicts 0.9 percent of women and 0.3 percent of men nationally. (2) And those numbers are only reported cases, not those who suffer in silence and secrecy. If there are seven billion people on the planet in any given year, then that percentage represents millions of unimaginable tragedies. An estimated twenty-four million in the U.S. alone. (3)

Has an eating disorder intruded into your world unannounced? Has your brain been hijacked, convincing you *skinnier is better* to the point you have lost interest in things that used to bring you joy and happiness? Or have you watched helplessly the decline of someone close to your heart? Did it hurt you deeply to watch him or her shrink away inch by inch, pound by pound? Are you terrified and scared and unsure what to do? Are you frozen with helplessness or overwhelmed with the confusing myriad of thoughts and feelings bombarding you? Do you wonder "What can I do?" and "Will this ever change?"

My heart, too, has felt these fears, and my head has pondered these questions. My world was shattered in an instant when I realized my son had developed an eating disorder. This illness came into my child's life and my awareness without warning or permission. It came out of left field and stripped my family of all we knew to be normal, replacing it with heaps of pain. I am a single mother of a teenage son who, after seven weeks of a scheduled *summer at Dad's*—an ocean away from me—went from smiling, healthy, happy, and energetic, to being malnourished, decaying, lethargic, and unable to eat or drink voluntarily. He waved goodbye the first week of June, and when he returned the last week of July, he was merely skin and bones, with a faraway look that suggested his body was just a shell for a vacant mind. I was in complete and utter shock. I can relate to how fearful you must be if you find this illness has entered your world. My action plan involved poring over every book I could find on the topic of eating disorders every waking moment. It was from a place of desperation that I sought assistance and hope.

In this book, you will find hope. You will discover that eating disorders have a course of onset; therefore, they have a course of reset. You will learn about the symptoms of anorexia and how this disorder affects an individual mentally, physically, socially, and emotionally. The difference between two of the more common eating disorders—anorexia nervosa and bulimia—will be explained, and you will glean a new understanding of malnourishment and how it can damage a person. And you will read of what one mom did to reverse these life-threatening symptoms and save her son.

I am the mother of two boys, ages eighteen and fourteen. I love my kids more than words can describe, and I am grateful for the chance to know them, love them, and parent them. I believe every life is of infinite value and worth, and it is a high calling and privilege to nurture those lives given to me by an all knowing loving Creator. I am a Christian and a believer in He who heals. I am a nationally board certified counselor, licensed mental health counselor, and a college level psychology instructor. I find human behavior incredibly complex and deeply enthralling, and I have been studying the field of psychology for nearly two decades. I am a counselor and a mom who is on a mission to thwart eating disorders and keep them from destroying lives, and I pray that by sharing our family's story, parents and other loved ones will be empowered to take action and fight for the health of those who cannot fight for themselves.

Perhaps as you are reading these pages and absorbing the words "eating disorder," you are mentally holding that term at arm's length with tweezers, afraid to let it get too close. You questioned your child's eating patterns, and you knew your child wasn't eating a lot for his or her age, but never in a million years did you imagine it was anorexia or another eating disorder. You worried and argued with your child about his or her weight being too low, and maybe, you even consulted with professionals to determine the level of concern warranted. Perhaps you even were told to seek counseling, but answers were elusive. Yet that knot in your stomach has not abated and your parent radar remains at high alert.

The accounts written in this memoir are the actual, unaltered experiences of my family unit. They were journaled within mere months of the events and, at times, written as events transpired. They are as truthful and detailed as one's recent memory can be, without the interference of time and intentional bias. My way of coping with the trauma I experienced as a mother watching her son dance with death was writing. It helped me stay grounded and in the here and now, while processing the unthinkable. My objective was to be authentic, honest, and transparent as I scribed what I saw, heard, felt, and witnessed.

Because this is a personal narrative from the parental perspective, the actions taken and advice given are not meant to replace or override the advice of medical personnel. I am not medically trained, and I do not hold the title of doctor, nutritionist, or psychiatrist. I cannot assure you the techniques used to help my son regain health will have the same result with your child, and I urge you to seek professional intervention and assistance in treating eating disorders because they are highly complex and individualized in nature. Different treatment modalities are available because eating disorders have varying causative forces. What worked for my family may not work for you, yet I do strongly believe these pages hold some valuable principles that will help guide and inform you.

In summary, although I cannot make predictive claims, I also cannot remain silent and not share what my family found helpful. The results have been miraculous, and full recovery from anorexia was indeed achieved. I do not know what the future holds for my son's health. No parent truly does. Yet I have full confidence and faith that he has become a new statistic...a survivor. One who beat the odds. And that did not happen by chance. Let the following pages walk you through that valley and up to the mountaintop where you can picture our unit of three holding hands held high in triumph and relief, fist-pumping the heavens. Now picture your family doing the same!

I want to be your advocate—your encourager, mentor, and accountability partner. I want this book to be a handkerchief for your heart and soul, and together, I assure you we can get through this issue and improve your child's life dramatically. Anorexia is a terrorist in the family! Swift and immediate action is required. Are you ready to begin? Are you ready to face the hijacker who stole your child's sanity? If so, let's get started.

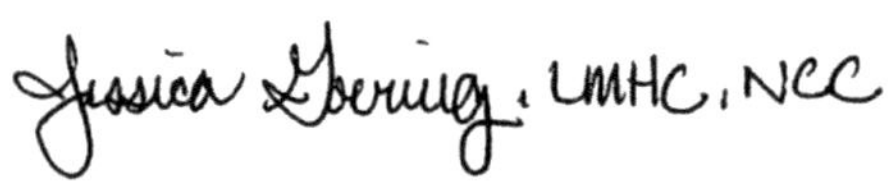

Note: The decision to print this memoir has come after much thought, prayer, and soul searching. I have contemplated "to print or not to print" for quite some time, believing transparency could help other families yet needing first and foremost to consider my son. Therefore, publishing was on hold for three years after this book was finished in order for him to reach adulthood and make his own informed decision about publicly telling our story. It is now being published with his permission and full blessing.

I fully realize that the story these pages holds is one that is very personal and raw. My professional conclusion is that it would be more damaging and destructive to align with the shame that some may attach to these experiences. Rather, I wish to stand for honesty, health, and healing which is summarized well in this quote by trauma expert Judith Lewis Herman:

> Remembering and telling the truth about terrible events are prerequisites both for the restoration of the social order and for the healing of individual victims. The conflict between the will to deny horrible events and the will to proclaim them aloud is the central dialectic of psychological trauma.

In an attempt to strike a balance close to privacy while refusing to aid and abet secrecy or shame, I have omitted my son's name from this writing and refer to him as "Brother" (capital B) in this account of his overcoming anorexia. Brother has been an affectionate term used to refer to him throughout his childhood since the innocent age of four when his younger brother entered the scene and looked up to his older counterpart with admiration. I hope this term doesn't confuse you, the reader, as the noun is used as a name replacement rather than a sibling position, although both are accurate.

Just as the body goes into shock after a physical trauma, so does the human psyche go into shock after the impact of a major loss.

— Anne Grant

CHAPTER 1

BRING THE PADDLES. I'M IN SHOCK.

So this is what Auschwitz survivors looked like. This can't be happening. My mind goes numb and my heart literally skips a beat—out of dread and pain—when I see him. Not the kind of heart skipping people want to experience—the kind that hits you like defibrillator paddles because the very life and soul of you has dematerialized into thin air.

I have just flown halfway across the world to get my boy after being told he won't eat and my ex-husband fears he has become anorexic. Somehow, this skinny, emaciated child in front of me is convinced he is fat. My ex-husband cautions me, "Don't talk to him about it, and don't hug him or he'll get upset." *Excuse me. This is my son...my heartbeat is in his heartbeat.* I can't understand this command, but I comply because that is what years of social conditioning have prepared me for. My parental barometer spins wildly as I notice everything about my son that isn't my son. It's as if the child I put on an airplane in June has been hijacked and a terrorist stands in his place...a look-a-like, just pretending and assuming his identity. Only even that is suspect because surely this can't be the same kid who smiled and hugged me as he prepared to board a flight for a summer visit with his dad a mere seven weeks ago.

Now he can't make eye contact, his face is gaunt, he can't stand still, he appears void of emotion, he paces constantly, he stands hunched over, he shivers uncontrollably, and he is covered in a jacket that despite its thick material, highlights shoulder bones protruding on a scrawny body. And it's the middle of summer! It's all I can do to stand. Suddenly, his cousins come out of the house to give hugs...apparently, they haven't been prepped, so they believe hugs are what cousins do! He tentatively and clearly painfully hugs back, but in a way that leaves his small cousins wondering what has changed. Something's wrong. He retreats to the house uncertainly as if he thinks he should go play, but has forgotten how. I cry loudly inside, but no one hears because I've been told not to show any emotion.

I go into crisis mode. This is the "fight-or-flight" moment you read about in textbooks. My body does it instinctively. Get help. Get help now. Get medical attention. He is dying and the world is letting it happen. I get on the phone and spend four painstaking days fighting insurance red tape to get my son into a specialized unit that will accept boys with eating disorders. Eating Disorder! Until this moment in time, eating disorders were something I had only read about, watched documentaries about, and seen shocking pictures of in magazines. I am in the mental health field, yet I am completely unprepared and unaware of how horrible this illness is and how quickly it can destroy someone I love. This healthcare hunt is a battle before the real battle, and I gear up for the long haul—an emotional reserve, so to speak.

On that shocking day, roughly two seconds passed between the moment I laid eyes on my child and the realization, beyond a shadow of a doubt, that he needed inpatient care for his malnourished state. Exactly 5,760 tortuous minutes passed between this awareness and adequate help. All the while I was left wondering whether my child would eat at all. Would he drink water? Would he stop breathing? Would he even wake up in the morning? Was his heart suffering damage, and would his organs shut down? Mind you, this time was spent in a frenzied state, making countless phone calls, exploring medical options, and embarking on a trip to the emergency room to check his vitals. He could not act for himself or think for himself! I believe his brain cells were devoid of nutrition long enough for his mental state to be compromised. He was a shell, and the vital life inside was being robbed of precious time.

That day, we tried in vain to eat out as an extended family. The cousins, ages five and seven, ordered food. Aunts and uncle did as well. We gathered in a holding pattern until we could get my son, Brother, life-saving intervention...yet in the meantime, we had to eat, right? This is what humans with appetites and economic resources do, right? Feel hunger, then eat. The seeming normalcy of that trip to a local restaurant will forever remain in my head. We were hungry. My emaciated child was hungry. But my son's brain would not allow him to partake. I ordered food for him anyway. I put the food in front of him. He cried; he panicked; he screamed; he trembled; he pushed away. And I cried with him. We tried again, unsuccessfully. He crumpled the food in his hands and ran away from the table. He refused even water. He was so upset that we had to leave the eatery. Another meal, and another minute, hour, and day when this child was starving in a time and place where food was plentiful. I wanted to scream.

What baffled me was that the insurance company didn't get it. Its employees sat in their air conditioned cubicles with a latte in one hand and a computer mouse in the other. At least, that was what I envisioned. Why wasn't it as simple as, "My son is starving to death; please admit him!"? Every phone call was precious time wasted, yet the insurance company seemed to be stalling over mere dollars and red tape. Outpatient. Inpatient. North region. West region. These were the terms tossed around in confusion since he was out of state when our crisis reached critical levels. It all seemed insane when I instinctively knew within seconds of our reunification that try as he might, he couldn't eat. Mentally, he couldn't do it. He had regressed, and in a thirteen-year-old form, he now had the capacity of a dependent and helpless two-year-old child...and this happened in seven weeks; how could that even be possible?

There was an odor. I don't have words to describe it. It was strange, decay-like, something I had never smelled before, and it was noticeable to me. It terrified me beyond words. I have always jokingly mocked my less than stellar sense of smell. Most things pass me unnoticed in this category. But not this time. July 27, 2013, a strange smell in my son's presence amplified my concern. This wasn't "normal," and my motherly instinct told me so.

And he followed me. He wouldn't walk next to me or in front of me, only behind me—and others. I found this terrifying and strange. It was as if he felt unworthy to walk alongside those around him. And that wasn't all. He trailed behind with a strange zigzag pattern that was eerie. He wouldn't or couldn't walk straight, and he compulsively mimicked his younger brother's actions. If his nine-year-old brother stood, then he stood. If his brother sat, then he sat. If his little brother would lie down, then he would lie down. If his little brother went to bed, then and only then would he allow himself to go down for the night. He inquired of his sibling frequently, "What do *you* want to eat?" and then made sure to get his brother food, all the while refusing any food himself. He was living vicariously through his brother as if self-care was not an option, so *other* care was paramount. It was so very hard to watch.

> ***TIP #1:*** *Pay attention to changes in your child's eating behavior, moods, interests, and appearance. They may or may not have an extreme debilitating onset like in our story, but they are signals for help nonetheless!*

Tearless grief bleeds inwardly.

— Christian Nevell Bovee

CHAPTER 2

AN OCEAN APART MAKES FOR AN INSIDIOUS START

Licensed Mental Health Counselor is my title. Well, my second title, given to me by the state. Mom is my first, given to me by God Almighty. Thankfully, in hindsight, I had some idea that things were going downhill for my oldest that summer based on communication with his father, whom he had gone to spend the summer with in New Mexico, as he had several times. His dad was concerned that since arriving at his home, Brother seemed to be eating less and less, was displaying an increasing amount of anxiety, and was pacing a lot. After a few weeks of concerning, yet vague communication, Brother's father suggested anorexia. Sight unseen, this possibility for my son was hard for me even to imagine. Complicating my confusion was the fact that I had not seen him on Skype, despite attempts, during these weeks because he had refused to sit in front of the computer when communicating with me. I had mentally chalked it up to normal adolescent separation and believed that although it was strange and atypical, perhaps he did not prioritize *seeing* Mom during his time with Dad.

It is mind-boggling to me how this change happened so quickly. Brother was eating normally before climbing the steps of that plane to leave our home in Hawaii. His food intake was typical when he first was at his dad's, including having snacks and sweets periodically between meals and at whim, as a healthy child does. And then, according to his father, Brother began eliminating items one by one from the menu. Much later, Brother disclosed to me that he essentially stopped eating one week after arriving at his dad's. He began declining snacks between meals and avoiding sweets. Then he started eliminating main course options. Pretty soon, he remained willing to eat only a small list of foods, including watermelon, cereal, pizza, chicken, apples, oranges, carrots, and peanut butter sandwiches. Everything else was considered taboo in his own mind. Then even those were being eliminated in part or totality. For instance, he would eat two to three chicken tenders at most, then suddenly refuse to eat more than one tender, and it had to have the breading peeled off. And the peanut butter sandwiches were no longer acceptable unless they were crust-less. Brother was becoming more and more stubborn in his starvation stance. He went from allowing himself to eat one slice of pizza to only two meager bites. One bowl of watermelon became three bites and then none. This decline was quick and insidious over the short summer weeks.

As my concern was increasing and his eating list was decreasing, I did some preliminary research and googled "eating disorder." The first webpage I encountered described an innovative technique called the *Maudsley Approach*, which essentially preached the importance of parental authority in the eating realm when working with children who are suffering from food restrictive behaviors. In other words, parents take back control over eating. This web search was no accident, but divine intervention, because it began a process of help unfolding in a series of miraculous events.

From that reading on, I urged my ex to make Brother eat *normal* portions (that sounds ignorantly simple, but it was all I could do from thousands of miles away) and then contacted the Eating Disorder Association of America (EDAA) to see what specialists were available on Oahu, Hawaii, where we lived. I intended to retrieve my son and place him in good, outpatient care while we figured out what was happening with him.

I had no idea of the real gravity of his situation. EDAA put me in contact with an angelic being, a therapist on the island who from that day on became our biggest supporter and lifeline in battling this life threatening monster. I dub her *Angel Ingrid*.

During an initial call, I shared a summary of my concerns with Ingrid and mentioned that my fear for my son had started with the results of a school physical Brother had undergone in New Mexico while at his dad's. I had been terrified when I heard the result of his weigh in...eighty-seven pounds. Although I wasn't aware of his exact weight when he left for his dad's, this number seemed shockingly low! His dad and I had then pursued counseling for Brother with a local provider in New Mexico, hoping to stop whatever *thing* was happening. After several weeks of counseling, Brother had only seemed to deteriorate emotionally and eat less. This deterioration included at least one incident when, according to my ex, Brother had hit himself in the face out of anger, leaving bruising. And, based on this information and more heartfelt sharing, Angel Ingrid startlingly recommended inpatient care and that I prepare myself for his condition being more dire than I had feared.

She was right. On the other side of the Pacific Ocean, the beginnings of what would soon be a dire medical emergency for our family were unfolding in Wisconsin. My two boys had been traveling with their father, my ex-husband, on a father/son trip across the continental USA. They started in New Mexico, headed to the Grand Canyon for some sightseeing, and then up north to their grandparents' cabin in the woods of Wisconsin. Typically, this destination is what I call "boy heaven." Picture a log cabin nestled in backwoods country with owls flying overhead and the purr of a motor on a pristine lake beckoning for fishing memories to be made. My boys loved spending time with their grandparents and have had many youthful, joyful moments there.

This trip was different, though. Dramatically different. Nothing takes the joy out of a vacation like starvation. Brother had no interest in anything his former self did, and his anxiety was reaching an all-time high.

In retrospect, this situation horrifies me because he was barely functioning, yet hiking parts of the Grand Canyon with *who knows what* degree of dehydration already setting in. Right before their stop at the canyon, I received communication from my ex that Brother had refused to eat anything at a fast food restaurant. My ex asked what he should do. Being 3,000 miles away and helpless, I begged him to apply tough love to whatever degree necessary to get compliance, and I stated I would be on the very next flight if he were not able to get Brother to eat. I wanted my son in the nearest emergency room or eating! I didn't understand what was happening!

Text after text came in rapid succession consisting of a back and forth between the two of us with Brother refusing to eat and my ex asking me what to do. I was getting very concerned so I called and asked to speak to my son, who was whimpering and crying in the background. Confused and fearful, I put on my firm parent voice and gave him the ultimatum: "Eat for Dad or I will come to get you on the next flight and there will be no Grand Canyon...rather a hospital bed." I was ready to pull out all stops to shift this trajectory. Brother's dad ended up compromising, allowing the meal to be eaten in the car en route because they were falling behind their travel schedule and needed to get to the next destination by nightfall.

This power struggle reached epic proportion before eventually ending in the tearful consumption of a few meager chicken nuggets, fast food size, with breading removed. I objected to acceptance of this on a parental level, but I was told I was not the one there and that was all that could be done at the time, so I accepted my inability to leap over the ocean and requested that Brother be given a supplemental nutrition shake at the next convenience store stop.

In my mind, the line in the sand was drawn and I was going to figure out what was happening with my child. He was no longer free to make his own eating choices. And he was no longer able to continue vacationing. I moved up my end of the summer flight date and planned to get my boy, while simultaneously arranging for inpatient admission for a child who, last time I had laid eyes on him, was healthy, happy, energetic, and *eating*.

In the course of communicating with professionals on the island of Oahu and preparing to intercept the children in Wisconsin, I thankfully learned from Angel Ingrid that Wisconsin boasted one of the nation's top hospitals for treating male adolescents with eating disorders.

This information about the hospital felt providential. Eating disorders afflict approximately .06 percent of the population (4) and of that number, only a small segment (10-15 percent of anorexic and bulimic sufferers) are male. Boys and men receive less help because of a preconception that this is a female specific disorder (3);

therefore, finding a qualified medical team to intervene was like finding a needle in a haystack. In fact, many treatment facilities deny male patients on the basis of gender alone. They are set up to receive female patients exclusively.

However, Roger's Memorial Hospital in Oconomowoc, Wisconsin, was a destination for male emaciated children worldwide and mere hours from Brother's grandparents' pristine lake. The possibility of pursuing treatment at Rogers was presented by Angel Ingrid before I even left Oahu and without even having laid eyes on my son. In my naivety about this illness, I had reassured myself, "At least he is eating." What! In hindsight I know he wasn't eating enough to keep a bird alive, much less a human, developing, pubertal child. This was ignorance and denial—and, sadly, my child's existence until I got on that winged bird that brought me face-to-face with my son's reality. When I arrived in Wisconsin and my eyes and nose and mind registered the damage in front of me, I knew Roger's was the only viable option.

In speaking with the intake specialist at this acclaimed hospital, I was told that Brother needed to pass an emergency department pre-screening to ensure he was healthy enough for admission into their inpatient ward. The absurdity of that hit me. But I went into autopilot and just followed instructions.

I can only imagine what thoughts ran through the mind of the nurse at the front desk when we walked into the Emergency Department that day: "What can I help you with?" she asked. There my son stood like a walking skeleton, which said more than I could explain anyway. My chocked up response was simply, "My son won't eat."

The staff took some background information and then proceeded to conduct a litany of tests, which, by the way, showed nothing except *clinical percentages*. This meant his liver could have 45 percent damage, but until it reached 85 percent, or whatever the magic threshold number was, would not register in standard medical tests. This knowledge was a blessing and a curse, as it left me terrified inside of what was around the corner, but certain that medical action was absolutely necessary.

Brother was dehydrated, so they hooked him up to fluids and proceeded to conduct an EKG. He struggled with this. You see, that exam involves lifting the shirt to place electrodes on the chest cavity. He protested and shed tears as the technician lifted his shirt briefly to place the metal plated circles. Meanwhile, I fought back gasps as I glimpsed the outlined shape of rib after rib in front of me. He barely moved other than to cover himself and try to hold back a noticeable tremble from the anxiety it caused him to be exposed. To see my son so vulnerable and helpless lying on that exam table was disturbing. As the test was conducted, my mind spun.

The results were mixed. The good news—no obvious permanent damage. The bad news—bradycardia (an abnormally low heartbeat). Official diagnosis given in that emergency department was anorexia. And the recommendation was for inpatient, acute care.

Then they let us leave. Leave! Go where? I didn't know what to do.

> ***TIP #2:*** *Take those changes in your child seriously and seek medical attention without delay. Don't be falsely reassured by the fact that your child is eating something, even meager portions. Ask the hard question: Is he or she eating enough for his or her developmental stage and age? Do your research. Seek experts in the field who work specifically with eating disorders!*

It is the peculiar nature of the world to go on spinning
no matter what sort of heartbreak is happening.

— Sue Monk Kidd

CHAPTER 3

INSIDE THOSE WALLS

We finally got the green light to admit Brother, and then I realized I was going to have to follow through with something that I hated to do, but had to do...drop my son off at a strange hospital with unknown doctors to treat an illness I could not believe he had. So, we drove. He had two blankets on him, a T-shirt, sweatshirt, and sweatpants, and he complained of being cold as we drove the two hours to Roger's Memorial Hospital. What was even more telling for me was what he did not do. He did not ask to stay home, he did not complain of going, and he did not protest. He needed help, and somewhere inside his nutritionally deprived brain, he knew it and was grateful.

When I type "he," I mean the person who is my child—not the "he" who attacked this boy and ravaged his brain....that persona I call *Terrorist Joey*. I'll introduce him to you later. But for now, I know that Terrorist Joey wanted to stay in control and certainly did not want to release his grip on this vulnerable child. But the dying child inside knew he could not fight this alone.

We found ourselves driving along a tree-lined road with beautifully landscaped grounds and immaculate, majestic brick buildings that seemed to say, "It's okay here."

We parked and grabbed Brother's suitcase, which held a quickly thrown together array of clothes I feared would not fit. The day prior, I had to rummage through old clothes that had no longer fit this child but were being called back into use through some cruel time warp where my teen who was supposed to be growing had shrunk.

As we walked through the sliding doors, I was relieved at the consistent appearance of the hospital's interior; it was clearly designed with great care, attention to detail, and upscale décor. Someone cared and, maybe, just maybe, I could trust that *someone* with *my everything*. As parents, we filled out the demanding paperwork, which essentially meant we would entrust our son to professionals who knew best. This need to trust others simultaneously terrified me and gave me great hope.

We walked with Brother to the locked ward where, once inside, you lose your "privilege" of normal, civilized society. No belts, no toys with strings, no shoes with laces, few personal belongings, no bags, no privacy....and no moms.

Brother's items were taken and searched, the drawstrings were cut out of his wardrobe, and he was given a hospital gown to wear. The whole time, I fought back tears and the impulse to run with him out the same door we had just come in, but that didn't seem to be a viable option if I wanted my son to eat again—an act so simple, taken for granted in the greater society, yet here was an unrivaled battle of wills. I noted Brother's legs, which looked like chopsticks, and his enlarged eyes and gaunt face. And then my eyes were drawn to his jaw and his bizarre teeth-clenching, which seemed to have appeared out of nowhere—along with the faint remaining evidence of facial bruising—and I concluded I could not run.

I stifled an internal urge to weep and walked with Brother down the hall to see where he would be staying indefinitely. We went through the motions of being interviewed by the social worker, meeting his nurse, skimming ward rules, and getting a schedule of what his days would entail. After he went through a brief physical exam, we were told his weight was a mere seventy-nine pounds.

And then we were expected to leave. This moment was heart-wrenching and one that will stay with me forever. Brother's dad and I told him we loved him and gave him a brief hug—which was all he seemed able to endure, and even that was still, rigid, and unreciprocated. Without emotion, he zigzagged to his room, and I walked into uncertainty.

We were able to visit the very next day and were given a report from his nutritionist and social worker. He ate breakfast. The three most blessed words I have ever heard! Strangely, though, he had told the social worker that "food was gross" and he had "never liked food." Weird since I had spent thirteen years with this special being—nursed him, fed him spoonfuls of his first vegetables and fruits, and helped him cut his meat until he could cut his own—had birthday parties with food galore and friend outings with pizza and all that kids call *yum*. Suddenly, his whole food recollection had been stolen and he insisted he hated food. How do you hate the very thing that keeps you among the living?

I guess that was Terrorist Joey again, the voice in his head that told him starvation was a good idea. What I have learned about anorexia, AKA *Terrorist Joey* in this writing, is that competing dialogues are occurring in the sufferer's mind. The voice of reason gets trampled by a barrage of negative self-talk and an assault of negative emotions that seem only to be relieved by food restriction.

For instance, my son would say, "I'm fat. I'm ugly. I'm stupid." These statements were verbalized periodically out loud but surely repeated in his mind like a broken record. Anorexia slipped in with false promises to make him feel *better* by controlling food and, therefore, giving him the illusion of control over these thoughts. The tragic paradox is that those who engage in this pattern of coping are trying desperately to control these *hard to feel feelings*, yet in the process, they lose all semblance of control as the illness takes over and the promise of *skinnier means happier* turns into a miserable existence. If existence at all! This disorder has the highest mortality rate of all mental illness diagnoses! Daniel Le Grange, Ph.D., director of the Eating Disorder Program at the University of Chicago informs, "Outcomes for AN are generally not optimistic. Only 44% of patients followed at least 4 years after the onset of illness are considered recovered, i.e., being within 15% of ideal body weight, one-quarter of patients remain seriously ill, and another 5% have succumbed to the illness and died. Other studies have reported mortality rates as high as 20% in chronically ill adults with AN." (5) And while these statistics reflect study done on the adult population, according to Dr. Erik Ulland, Brother's psychiatrist and Medical Director of Inpatient Child and Adolescent Services at Rogers Memorial Hospital, "If Eating Disorders (ED) continue, a teen becomes an adult with an ED unless it is treated or resolves 'naturally'—which is cause to cringe to think of something so potentially dangerous being left to resolve naturally." There was no simple cure, or *snap out of it and eat mantra*. Armed with this knowledge, as a parent and mental health professional, I knew we were in a life or death fight with Terrorist Joey. And we had to win. The alternative was not an option.

For some, this illness is characterized by a perfectionistic belief that one is achieving *health* by only eating the bare minimum required to live. It is a deadly delusion. The problem is that anorexics are overconfident in their ability to toe the line, and many succumb to death despite their desire to stay above the lifeline. Because the decline is largely hidden internally in the bones, the organs, the bloodstream, the muscles, the tissues, and the cells, depending on the severity of their food restriction and/or purging behaviors, they can appear healthy to the average person, yet be inching near their own graves. Just as one's brain is likely to be overconfident in driving ability when drunk or texting, so the anorexic or bulimic is equally unable to determine how little to eat and still be able to wake up the next morning.

Miscalculations are fatal. They can have a damaging cumulative effect on the body, and the effect they have on the central nervous system, muscular-skeletal system, organs, heart, brain, and the like is severe. Brother was on this death march and quickening his pace over the summer—to a degree unknown to me at the time.

Something changed for my son that first day of inpatient care. Thankfully, an outside voice was now competing with the inside voice that promised "starvation is better." Now, adults and caregivers in his world were saying, "Eat, or you have to stay here in a strange place away from family and all that you know and care about." And the supportive voices challenged his internal dialogue, targeting the fear at the root of the eating behaviors. He sat in Cognitive Behavioral Therapy (CBT) groups that taught him some of the thinking errors that contributed to his depression, anxiety, and the drastic decline in his food intake. These professionally led groups provided reality testing by pointing out the true state of his life and how the thinking errors—personalizing, all-or-none thinking, catastrophizing, generalizing, mind-reading, and labeling—were counterproductive and unfairly contributing to his self-destruction. He was also required to participate in confidence-building activities and individual counseling sessions, which provided alternative perspectives and experiences to counter the internal chaos. One specific reframe that helped Brother was Dr. Ulland's explanation of "health" in a way that countered his fragmented mind's definition. Dr. Ulland explained to Brother the medical benefits and longevity statistics of having slightly *more* substance rather than substantially *less*. This message wasn't accepted by Brother at face value and embraced, but it gave momentary pause to the snowballing vice of anorexia.

Being in this setting jumpstarted Brother's eating and, in my opinion, was one more indication of The Miraculous Healer in his midst. Throughout the duration of his stay, he ate all his meals. This may come across as being an easy thing, but I can assure you it was not! It would be simplistic and inaccurate to assume that he just stopped eating and could then just restart eating again with some semblance of his old self. His compliance was evident, although the manner in which this took place was bizarre.

He would eat, but it was as if he had to relearn this basic skill. Meals in the hospital took an hour on average, and he seemed to savor each bite, or resist each bite; it was hard to tell. Each bite was methodically lifted from plate to mouth, yet it was strange and robotic. The person Brother was inside this body shell seemed to have checked out and left the space vacant. His face was expressionless, he barely spoke, and his demeanor was very reserved.

We were instructed not to talk about food but just be with him. So that is what we did.

It's hard to talk about the sports channel when your son is on a locked hospital ward being told exactly what to eat, when to eat, where to sleep, and, essentially, how to exist. And the space his body fills on this planet was eerily small and a constant illustration of his near-death status. Things in general went in slow motion; he would talk slow, walk slow, and think slow. He was sensitive to touch and would avoid physical contact with family or staff. He could not even give a high-five, as if the sensation of touch required was physically painful. He rarely sat down because he admitted to his doctor that it hurt—his bones protruded from his backside. When he did sit, he could not or would not lean back. He paced or stood upright constantly and seemed anxious *all* the time. He was taking cold showers only, which I feared was self-punishment, and he refused to wear his contacts.

Throughout Brother's treatment, this phenomenon seemed to be explained by his lack of desire to *see* himself. Despite his extreme thinness, he believed himself to be obese. He felt fat and was certain he was fat. Anorexia is a thought-based illness of distorted perception. *Distorted* meant he did not see the same image that you and I see. His mirror experience was like looking in a carnival mirror that displays an image that doesn't match reality. For example, a body shape that is actually skeletal and gangly appears round and plump. The visual field brings in data, which is processed inaccurately in the brain's perceptive areas; because the round image is what the sufferer truly sees, he cannot be reasoned into thinking otherwise. In fact, he thinks everyone around him is wrong or overtly lying! For Brother, even a slight glance at his own reflection would cause him great distress. He refused to open the curtains in his room because he did not want to see his reflection in the window pane. Most of the time, he declined to use electronics for the same reason. He had not had a haircut all summer, so his hair had grown into a tangled mess, to which he seemed oblivious. His nails needed cutting and were filthy. He was generally disheveled in appearance. His whole demeanor suggested, "Just let me shrink away."

Ambivalence was his frequent companion until approximately midway into his hospitalization. At that point, he began to cry and say he wanted to leave. This reaction compounded our difficulty in making him stay. Then another child got admitted onto the ward and was discharged one day later. Brother pleaded with us to take him home because "she got to" and "her parents took *her* home." I so desperately wanted to, but this moment in time required a powerful act of tough love, and tough love needed to prevail. So I told him I loved him and would be back to see him tomorrow, and that is how our lives spun in a strange manner for eight entire days.

I began to pore over eating disorder books to understand this better while he participated in counseling groups, met with his psychiatrist, and was monitored physically. He saw children like himself, some with feeding tubes in their mouths for forced intake, and gratefully, he talked about not wanting "that."

In one of his therapeutic activities, Brother was asked to draw his *safe place*. He drew a beautiful ocean wave. In addition, he talked frequently of his love of surfing and, although he had lost interest in almost everything else, he retained this passion. Not only did he retain it; he seemed abnormally desperate for it. And this was surprising because he had only lived in Hawaii for six months before his summer visit; surfing was a new interest that I hadn't known to be so important to him already.

Instinctively, I knew in my heart he needed to go home—his Hawaii home—and he needed to be in healing waters. That was his place of comfort and happiness, and I was determined to help him get there. He was considered eligible for release because he was following his meal plan and had gained four pounds in eight days, which was extremely encouraging. The clinical staff recommended residential living on campus to continue his treatment—potentially for months.

Parenting requires an insane amount of decision making! I evaluated all the options and discussed them with his father, yet felt firmly in my heart, after listening to my child, that he needed to be back in Hawaii. My trepidation at that time was, "But would he eat for me?" This was unknown and unchartered territory since Terrorist Joey had unpacked in his head.

Brother was discharged on a Wednesday and I gave him the option of flying back to Hawaii Friday or Saturday. Paradoxically, with very little decisive power left in his brain, this decision seemed easy for him. Friday.

So, I purchased return tickets to Hawaii for Friday.

The next two days were a trial period of sorts. I had a discussion with him that discharge was contingent on him eating, and if he went back to refusal of food and water, then I would, out of love and concern, be forced to readmit him. He needed this! The fight was in his head, and I chose to take it from him. Therefore, "Should I eat or not eat, and what kind of food will I allow myself to eat, and how many calories does it have?" could be trumped by the adult voice saying, "You will eat for me or for the hospital staff. That is your only choice."

The sense I had from my research and short exposure to this horrible illness was that when given the choice, the sufferer will *always* pick starvation or minimal consumption. Taking the choice away helped immensely.

Armed with a meal plan compiled by the hospital's nutritional staff, we stayed with my brother, who lived nearby, for those two days. The meal plan concept was strange for a mother who up this point in childrearing just fed her children and allowed them to respond to their appetites regarding portion control. Now, I had to measure, count, and plan every morsel that entered my child's body.

Ensure became a new vocabulary word for our family. The hospital policy was that if eating disorder patients did not eat or did not complete their meals, they were given Ensure...you know, those calorie laden nutritional supplements. Apparently, he was not a fan of Ensure, so this worked to his treatment advantage. Ensure became ammunition for me, and I armed myself with a six pack of it!

Those two days went by in a blur and my anxiety rose. Now *my* thoughts were pricked with self-doubt. "Could *I* do it?" This child needed around-the-clock monitoring. He would only eat when it was required of him through adult supervision and enforcement, and even then, he required monitoring for at least an hour afterward to prevent purging behaviors, which were feared at this point and could not be given an opportunity to rear their ugly head.

To complicate matters, his meals were taking longer and longer to complete—one to two hours on average. He was given three meals a day, plus three snacks, and this totaled six eating sessions a day with the snacks taking nearly an hour as well.

Enforcement of his eating was now a full-time job—an approximately seven to nine hour a day commitment. As a single parent, I was working full-time at one job and part time from home at another, so I didn't see how I could balance work with his eating; it didn't seem humanly possible in my head. But Brother wanted to be in the ocean. His artwork said so. His weakened voice said so. When given the choice between flying to Hawaii on Friday or waiting one more day with extended family, he chose Friday. My job was to sort through what he needed, and listening was my tool of choice.

I suppressed my urge to quit my job, stay with family, and nurture my boy back to health on the mainland. An inner quiet, calming presence encouraged me to go back to the ocean, his safe place. I had to find a way to do that.

Have you ever had to make the decision to go through with something that seemed completely impossible and you had no idea how to make it work? That was my reality in that moment. As a parent, I have never been as frightened, confused, overwhelmed, and scared as I was getting on that plane on August 9, 2013.

I literally bit my lip so I would not weep uncontrollably in front of my children. I can still taste the fear when I recall that moment. We went through security, the boys said goodbye to their dad, and I realized with trepidation that I was alone in this. I was *terrified* to be alone in this.

Sadly, I had no idea how accurate my prediction was. And, bam, the first hiccup came in the security line. Yep, I was smuggling on Ensure! I was told to relinquish the liquid gold or endure an embarrassing pat down. Option number two, please. Really, what options did I truly have? It was a small price to pay to have calorie backup on the flight over the Pacific Ocean with a child who might or might not eat for me.

My emotions that flight were a strange brew of anxiety, edginess, concern, sadness, and worry, sprinkled with gratitude. Would the miles between Brother and the hospital cause him to regress? Would the brothers ever play together again? Would I ever see my son smile again? Would Terrorist Joey try to unpack and reside in our home for good? Would I have to quit my job? Would I be able to afford that? Would we have to move? Would I truly be able to work two jobs and give this child twenty-four-hour care—which he needed?

And the scariest question and deepest fear—would he die?

And if he survived, would he suffer endlessly?

Going home away from extended family support and treating Brother's illness seemed completely incompatible, yet vitally necessary. Doubts assailed me, and yet the gratitude of a child four pounds heavier than when I first laid eyes on his frail form comforted me and provided some hope to reach for.

My faith is an anchor in my life. Several times in my life, I have acted in faith, based on my intuitive sense that I had to leap into the unknown to save myself and/or my children. This time was no different. I believed intensely and with great conviction that Brother needed to return to Hawaii, and that was the only reason I was able to board that flight. In hindsight, this peace was an arrow lighting our path, and I am grateful to my God for that direction in a time of overwhelming uncertainty.

> ***TIP #3:*** *Eating is non-negotiable! Take the option away. The actions required to accomplish this tactic will vary, but the importance of reestablishing authority is vital.*

When we love, we are courageous; and courage has nothing to do with being fearless, it's about being willing to experience fear, even dread, to do what we must, without guarantee of outcome.

— Vanna Bonta

CHAPTER 4

TAKEOFF INTO UNCHARTED TERRITORY

Other kids laughed or cried, parents talked, people plugged into various entertainment devices, and stewardesses offered the usual peanut and drink options. I took the food and drink graciously and then thought, *Now what?*

I looked at my oldest son, covered in sweats from head to toe and wrapped in another thick fleece blanket borrowed from family for this challenging flight experience. Other passengers had on light clothing, anticipating Hawaii's warm climate. Brother was shivering continuously and complaining of being cold, and meanwhile, I couldn't stop thinking, *I have to wake up from this nightmare!*

Instead, I got my child's attention and firmly told him he would have to eat now. He complied, but this seemingly small task took forty-five minutes from start to finish. Just peanuts and a drink! Sometime during that flight, I had a flashback to comments I had made occasionally as I parented my children. In the past, I would jokingly and lovingly say that they were growing up too fast and I wanted to keep them around forever. "Where is the pause button?" I would banter. Now, with regret, I wondered whether this innocent and playful message had been misinterpreted—perhaps my child wanted to stay a child, and now at the intersection of childhood and adolescence, he was subconsciously trying to thwart this milestone. I looked at my son next to me and asked directly, "Are you afraid to grow up?"

To my surprise, he actually nodded affirmatively. This afforded me a chance to share with him that growing up is a wonderful thing and what all parents want for their children. Selfishly, we parents will miss the cuddles and the part about being needed, but we want our children to have their own lives and the freedom and adventures that growing up give.

Brother gave a brief nod, and we continued our journey in relative silence. Talking requires energy, and he was on his reserve tank.

Several hours later, we landed and experienced a layover. It was time for our first meal away from the accountability of hospital staff or the support of extended family. We were alone in a crowd of faces. I set the boys down at a table and scanned the menu, finding a meal I thought had sufficient calories for Brother. Then I placed the order. Having a meal felt like a monumental task. One with lots of risk and no room for error. Treatment now required *all* food provided to this child must be eaten.

His meals were five course. All of them. He was no longer given a choice as to what he wanted. I had ordered for him a full order of buffalo chicken wings, celery, corn on the cob, biscuits with butter, and milk to wash it down. Dessert to follow.

We had two hours for me to ensure my malnourished child consumed enough calories to make it through the next leg of the flight. I also knew I had to use this time to make plans for treatment upon arrival on the island. I frantically made phone calls to providers, trying to align a task force that would be ready to help immediately, and yet I didn't want to expose my children to this behind the scenes work, so I had to find a place where I could observe them (and make sure Brother didn't dump the food!) while also having privacy for sharing a summary of his condition.

I walked a few feet away and, hiding in the crevice of a storefront opposite the eatery, did my best to manage two priorities. Pressure was high because I was only able to take one more week off, unpaid, before risking losing my job (I had already taken two to accommodate travels and his inpatient stay), and if I lost my job, so would he lose his opportunity for *ocean therapy.* Time was a luxury of which Brother and I had little. Since the hospital experience had effectively kick-started his compliance with authority directed eating, my thought process was that if he continued to experience this kind of intervention uninterrupted, he would essentially be forced to recover. I truly believed that he had to be required to eat and could not make this choice of his own accord because of the effects of malnourishment on his brain. The latent worry was that if he were allowed to regress back to food avoidance, his chances of staying on the track of eating and recovery would be short-lived. Essentially, I saw a window of opportunity to reverse this!

I finalized plans with a nutritionist, psychiatrist, and medical provider while watching my child like a hawk. It took the entire two hours before he was finished eating and we could rush to the connecting flight.

I was exhausted before the next plane touched down and yet now that we were back on the island, my mission was to re-nourish a malnourished child. Grocery shopping would have been necessary regardless, but under these conditions, it became my utmost priority.

The task also created a quandary of sorts. Should I take a child who has bouts of anxiety at the sight of food to the grocery store, or leave that same child home at risk of vomiting and exercising excessively—which looks like hours of zigzag pacing? This was one of his most tell-tale symptoms, erratic pacing—either intentionally to burn calories because he thought he was fat, or the result of a malnourished mind fixated on food but unable to consume willfully. Think how anxious you get when you miss one meal! Now multiply that by the many meals that Brother shortchanged himself on this summer. You can be sure his anxiety was visible. Hmmm. Had I had the third option of cloning myself, I would have walked into that lab. But instead, I chose the lesser evil and dragged my ill child into aisle after aisle of canned and packaged trauma.

Calorie counting was Terrorist Joey's friend and my enemy. So I instructed Brother to ignore all labels and keep his hands off all food goods and remain at my side like a toddler. Then I had to revise completely my shopping paradigm and look for high calorie foods rather than low fat. What mom does this? What conscientious food manager of a home actually goes aisle by aisle and thinks, "Hmm, let's see; what is the fattiest food I can buy? What is the highest calorie drink I can purchase? What is the most caloric sweet that takes the shortest time to eat?" I told myself to hurry on Brother's account, but the reality was that I had to think! I had to think how to manage his 3,500 calorie a day meal plan and make it out of this market mentally intact with two children in tow.

I sneakily checked labels and slid items into the cart, while cautioning my son to avert his eyes as I did so. Nope, this one says *low fat*. Put it back. That one says *skim*. Run away. This one says *fat free*. What is wrong with society? That one says *100 calories*. Try again. This one touts *low calorie*. "I want FAT!" my mind screamed. With my cart full of medical supplies (aka "food") and cases of Ensure by bulk, I survived that shopping excursion, and with relief, I slid into the driver's seat and put the car in gear. Onward to home. To the fridge. To the table. To the mouth. In that order. Food, check. Next target to conquer, school staff.

Thus began what I call *rally the forces*. Anyone in Brother's circle who would be able to fill in while I worked was a necessary recruit! In addition to the professionals involved, I needed his school on board, as well as the adults in his life who would provide before and after school care. Which by the way, due to having only lived in Hawaii a short time before his falling ill and even then having just relocated to another part of the island, meant it was a new school so the staff had no working knowledge of this child or what he was like in a healthy state. And to top it off, he had just spent his first week of the school year in a locked, inpatient psychiatric ward halfway across the world.

I called the school counselor and requested a meeting. One of the scariest things was expecting this kid to go to school. *School* was a six letter horror movie in my mind that equated to half a day of unsupervised time for Terrorist Joey to run amuck. Its obstacles included starvation torture, dehydration, mirrors all over, kids who taunt (especially when you wear a sweatshirt in Hawaii and walk in a zigzag pattern unable to look people in the eye as you clench your mouth uncontrollably and unconsciously).

To my great relief, the staff members at his school listened. They heard my concerns, and in an act of unprecedented assistance with this illness, they offered to place him on a 504 plan, which in the state of Hawaii is for disabled students and allows for specific accommodations to ensure needs are met during school hours (Section 504 Subpart D Hawaii Law and Regulations).

Hallelujah! I felt some hope seep in with that three digit number. The counselor, dubbed *Angel Angie*, agreed to supervise Brother's eating at lunch and also to pull him out of class for the required morning snack time, per his individualized meal plan. This was unheard of in the community. I have spoken to many parents with similarly diagnosed children who have not received this kind of extra assistance. I am convinced this support was paramount to his rapid recovery, in contrast to many who suffer for decades. It guaranteed he would be given food and water during the day, which his brain would not allow him to self-initiate, and it would prevent any intense hunger cravings from having the chance to develop and, therefore, increase his restrictive impulses.

Additionally, it meant he would be monitored for thirty minutes post-eating to minimize his urges to purge. Binging and purging are behaviors of the sister illness, bulimia. Both disorders involve a deep-seated fear of *fat*. Whereas anorexia is characterized by food restriction and starvation, bulimia is a disorder characterized by eating binges and subsequent purging of calories from the body in an attempt to avoid weight gain. This can be done by vomiting, laxatives, diet pills, or excessive exercising. Brother had been oriented to the purging process in the hospital. Questions about binging and purging were asked at intake and every day in the hospital thereafter. According to his inpatient psychiatrist, Erik Ulland, MD, children with restrictive type eating disorders are at high risk to turn to bulimia and purging methods as their illness progresses. The risk is as high as 9 out of 10, for adults who do not receive treatment. Dr. Ulland informs "The Cognitive Behavioral Treatment formulation suggests that eating disordered individuals are focused on weight, shape, and/or health *and* the mistaken belief that they can control any aspect of this *long term*. The reality is that if the illness proceeds long enough, an anorexic will eventually begin the binge purge cycle, become on average slightly overweight, and out of control with eating behaviors. This must be a horrible reality when before the anorexic felt in control and was at a lower weight. Without treatment, if anorexics survive the illness long enough, they are most likely to lose control—even the most consistent of them. With successful treatment, anorexic adults tend to stabilize at the low end of their ideal bodyweight range. Also, it's important to note that probably the most dangerous point is if and when severely underweight people begin the binge purge cycle. They are more likely to suffer medical mortality at that lower weight with fluctuations in fluids—cardiac arrhythmias." Because of this scary realization, I viewed the school staff as resources to help stand in the gap and restrict access to purge as a vitally important strategy toward nipping Terrorist Joey's momentum. In other words, preventing the binge/purge cycle from even starting seemed part of that window of opportunity to hit "reset" rather than increase Terrorist Joey's grip on this fragmented mind.

Because their anxiety over eating has nowhere to go, sufferers often engage in secretive and destructive ways of avoiding calorie digestion. My son was at the point where he believed even water was unacceptable consumption, and therefore, he refused even this simple life-saving energy source. In fact, while he was hospitalized, one of his daily goals was to consume just one whole eight-ounce bottle of water, and he would baby this, hardly touching it unless prompted. During visiting hours in the late afternoon, I would worry as I noticed barely a tablespoon gone from the water line.

This goal was incrementally increased, yet he remained avoidant of all liquid as well as solid nourishment. The only barrier between him and starvation and complete dehydration was adult authority. During the course of bringing Brother home, I had also been in contact with *Angel Kirsten*, my dear friend who agreed to watch him before and after school; she was on board with his medical nutritional needs and willing to enforce expectations in that environment as well. Without this wraparound care, I do not doubt that I would not be writing this book with the same ending.

That first week back in Hawaii, I did not return to work; rather I made it my job to be a visible presence every morning and every afternoon at Brother's school. I introduced myself to the health aide, the administration, the secretary, Brother's homeroom teacher, and the lunch lady. I smiled with great flair to all, wishing I could lay down a welcome mat for my son as he bravely entered this new school in a condition where he was unable to engage socially with anyone.

I probably annoyed the secretarial staff a great deal, but it was par for the course. I wanted them to know me because I was scared to return to work and delegate this very important mission to strangers. I brought Brother his morning snack and lunch daily, and I sat with him in the health aide's office. The plan was for the school counselor to assume this duty upon the start of the second week, when I had to return to work, and until then I was going to set the standard. Just as my world was unprepared for anorexia, so apparently was everyone else's. The health aide, kind man as he was, made well intentioned comments as I would open up the sack lunch contents.

"Oh, a turkey sandwich and Oreos. Every kid likes those. Surely he will eat that." Understandable comments, but our "surely" didn't exist anymore. The only *sure* thing I was aware of anymore was that I *sure* better make *sure* my son eats or he will *surely* die. So I smiled outside and grimaced inside and mumbled something to the effect of "Eating is very hard for him right now."

I wanted to explain Brother's condition to people in order to gain their support and monitoring help, but at the same time, I wanted to hide the problem to protect his reputation and privacy. I feared his entering a new school and being dubbed the weird kid, the one who walks funny, or the one who starves himself, or the one with anorexia. You see, as far as I was concerned, this anorexia thing was an unwelcome squatter in his life. An intruder. I didn't want him labeled, and I sure didn't want him to be known as Terrorist Joey going forward.

But these people had no baseline to work from. They had never met my child before this day. They couldn't identify the imposter because they didn't know the real boy. They had no idea that he didn't usually look this sick and he didn't usually walk this way. He didn't usually clench his mouth awkwardly and have a far-away look in his eyes. They didn't know that he normally smiled at people and had a great sense of humor and played sports every chance he could. They didn't know that he had the biggest heart and was academically gifted. They didn't know that he historically had gotten in the food line with his peers and said, "Please" and "Thank you" as he received his school meal and sat down with friends, perfectly capable of eating until his stomach was content. These people didn't know Brother! They were meeting Terrorist Joey walking in Brother's frail frame, and I was his mother but now also his school representative.

These staff members did amazing things, having no or very little understanding of anorexia. His homeroom teacher gave me his direct line so I could check on Brother at any moment. His principle volunteered to eat with Brother when the school counselor was not available. The health aide offered us the private space of his office and gave much needed encouragement to me as I passed through the school's doors more frequently than I had thought humanly possible. He talked surf with Brother, which was about the only thing that seemed to make Brother smile or be willing to converse with anyone. The school security officer would observe him and give me a report when I asked. Typically, it was more of the same. "He walks alone. Sits alone. Acts strange. And doesn't talk to other kids. But he stays out of trouble."

I had several hoops to jump through so I made it my business to hike up my skirt and *jump*. Brother was required to have his picture taken per school policy and wear an ID on his lapel during school hours. It was part of the uniform. No big deal for 99.9 percent of the student population. But for my son, this was triggering. You see, with anorexia, the sufferer truly does not *see* the image the rest of the public sees. The image Brother saw was still distorted. He glanced at his school picture and cried. Then he threw it away. And this was less than a week after release from an inpatient eating disorder unit where he was too thin to sit without pain!

I looked at that picture and cried too! But for vastly different reasons! Thankfully, the school showed some initial leniency, and as time wore on, we compromised by having Brother wear the ID backwards, image facing inward. This seemed more manageable for him.

In addition to the required ID, the school uniform also consisted of his school's branded T-shirt, mixed with bottoms of personal choice. Thankfully, the school was lax in this area also because he refused to wear a T-shirt alone and shivered even under a thick pullover sweatshirt. Rather than expecting him to wear the trendy clothes I had naively purchased for the upcoming school year, I sent him to school each day in elastic banded athletic shorts that would, hopefully, stay up and not fall off. No longer did I worry whether he would be fashionable enough to fit in. Now I worried about his pants falling off and how to avoid his being a target for bullying! When your child loses his health, everything else that used to matter—matters no more.

In my quest for recruits on island for Project Heal Brother, it crossed my mind to contact the Hawaii University Football Team quarterback, Taylor Graham. Brother had always looked up to athletes and had an exceptional amount of admiration and respect for this particular young man since he was not only accomplished on the field, but he also attended our church and displayed good character and spiritual strength.

My sons had been blessed to play dodge ball with Taylor earlier that year on Easter Sunday, and I knew they had felt special and important that day because of Taylor. I hoped that maybe this quarterback could reach a part of Brother that was still listening. And I knew Taylor could eat! Football players have to consume a lot of fuel given the extreme amounts of energy they expend on the field and in the gym.

I emailed Taylor. By the Grace of God, he responded. And with a giving and caring heart to boot! He admitted that anorexia was not something he understood well or had tactics to help with, but he cared. He cared about my son. And he wanted to get to know

Brother. He wanted to be his friend. That sounds simple, but it was a big deal. Taylor began texting my son regularly, encouraging and lifting him up.

I will never forget the first time he texted Brother. You see, at this point, Brother had zero social interest. He cared about nothing outside of the drive to be skinny. He had put aside all thoughts of interacting with people, especially new peers, or even conversing with anyone outside a very small circle of people he deemed emotionally safe. He also rejected his phone with the exception of one day when he noticed a new message on the screen. As he read it and Taylor's name registered, I saw the biggest smile cross his face since anorexia had invaded his brain.

He actually smiled. A genuine outward sign of internal joy. It was so refreshing to see that I felt a surge of hope. Taylor kept in touch with Brother regularly throughout the next few months. Brother still rejected his phone and rarely had the energy or care to text back, but when I brought Taylor's texts to his attention, he read each message. And those messages mattered. It mattered that this athlete took time to text him about his travels, his games, and his life. It was another proxy for Brother to live through until he could reclaim his own space on this planet. I am forever grateful to Taylor for how he cared about my son.

Brother's meal times increased. His seven to nine hour time commitment to food increased to roughly ten to twelve! Which meant so did the commitment of the adults in his world. I am not sure what happened, but the more time passed post hospital release, the longer it seemed to take him to eat. His eating was regressing. He would take bites that were shockingly small or startlingly large and was oblivious to where the food landed—on his face, nose, neck, cheek—anywhere in range seemed acceptable. It was literally like watching a two-year-old try to manage a fork.

I don't know how to explain this, but somehow, his self-awareness was stifled. After *rally the troops week*, I started back to work and we entered *time havoc week*...okay, let's be honest, time havoc *months*. Our days usually started around four a.m. since I had to get myself ready for the day before preparing him a hot breakfast and then sitting with him as he consumed it slowly, bite by tiny bite, to guarantee he had one complete meal in his belly unpurged before he started his school day.

We had to leave our house by 6:15 in order for me to take the boys to Angel Kirsten's house, so she could monitor Brother before school while I took my place in the line of Honolulu traffic. Then I would start my work day and anxiously await word from Brother's counselor on how he was eating and managing during snack and lunch. I prepared bags of snacks for two weeks at a time and stocked the school health aide's fridge for the midmorning monitored snack. I hand-packed his lunch daily to ensure it met the calorie expectations of his meal plan and directly handed it to my friend in the morning when I dropped him off. She then hand-delivered it to an adult member of the school staff, who would hand it off to the counselor. Whew. Massive coordination and organization that was literally lifesaving in intent! This happened quickly and smoothly, and if it had not been seamless, it would have allowed countless opportunities for Terrorist Joey to increase his power.

However, Brother knew his food was *never* solely in his control until an eyewitness was available to confirm or deny his ingestion of the contents. And even then, he was watched so it would stay there! I believe this provided his brain a sense of relief and resignation to following the treatment plan.

The counselor emailed me a daily status report, which greatly helped us align tactics and make sure consistency was part of Brother's day. She brought to my attention his excessive napkin use. Really! Of course, why not? He began obsessively and compulsively using napkins to wipe away any residue of food on the corners of his mouth—to the point that the wiping caused sores. And he began to pick at the food remnants in his teeth with great care and ritual. So the decision was made to take away his napkins until the meal was completed; then he was allowed only a solo tissue to clean up. He was also instructed to stop picking at his teeth. This restriction—like many others that resulted from his new, strange, obsessive, and compulsive tendencies—caused an emotional meltdown. His anxiety over forced eating was trying to filter its way out however possible, and each time the boat sprung a leak, the professionals and I tried to plug the hole. The *hole*, however, looked different each time.

> ***TIP #4:*** *You don't have to do this alone. Get everyone on board who can respect confidentiality in your child's world and still be powerful accountability help to reinforce the meal plan. Eyes and ears can be helpful in all settings throughout the child's day. Don't leave gaps in coverage.*

After all, when a stone is dropped into a pond,
the water continues quivering even after
the stone has sunk to the bottom.

— Arthur Golden

CHAPTER 5

MALNOURISHMENT ALTERS BRAIN CHEMISTRY

To help you understand a day in the life of a malnourished child, let's rewind to the process of just getting out of the house in the morning. I would wake up and get myself ready so I would be fully available when Brother woke because he needed constant monitoring and prompting. I would prepare a full breakfast, including all tiers of the food pyramid, in a one-stop shop. Then I would wake him up and tell him breakfast was ready.

After this momentous task, Brother would sit and stare into a far-away place, unable to self-initiate anything. I would tell him to start eating just so he would make the arm motions necessary to grab the utensils. He was in such a mental fog that he seemed to need directions for all actions of normal daily living. I would explain to him that he needed to brush his teeth. He would respond and go do so, but he would not stop unless I told him it was time to stop.

One morning, I recall forgetting to tell him to stop because I was distracted by another task. He continued to brush for over ten minutes, until I realized what was happening. I felt horrible. He would stand by the door, unsure what to do, until I would say, "Now go change your clothes" or "Put on your sandals" or "Put in your contacts" (which was now a self-care requirement), or "Open the door and walk down the stairs and get in the car."

Driving him to school was another obstacle. If I looked at him, he would cry. If I said the wrong thing, he would cry. I had to be careful and emotionally prepare myself to check for traffic if I needed to turn left or right. He would misinterpret any glance back as looking at him, and then he would begin to cry and bemoan, "See, I am fat!" or "I'm so fat you can't see around me!" He would only sit in the rear passenger seat because from any other position in the car, he could see his reflection in the car mirrors and would meltdown in panic. When I would pull into the driveway of Angel Kirsten—my friend who had graciously agreed to provide before and after school care—he would sit, seemingly unsure of what to do next. When I would prompt him, he would get out, walk up the driveway, and go inside to stand. Just stand. Sometimes, he would awkwardly stand very near Angel Kirsten so as to stalk the hand towel in her kitchen, which he wanted for wiping the corners of his mouth. If the hand towel were taken from him or access to it was blocked, he would pace. Often, before I could even reach work, I would get some sort of communication that he was struggling. This was horrendous to walk through and I was outside his head! Imagine the pain and turmoil inside. *You are fat. Obese. Disgusting. Ugly. Huge. A disgrace. Stupid. Worthless. Incapable.* I imagine this was the broken record he constantly heard replaying in his head. At least, from his actions and moods, I could confidently infer it.

Brother didn't know what to do with himself and didn't have any of his previous interests, with two exceptions: surfing and Legos. So I surrounded him with both. Legos in his room (I brought back an entire suitcase full from the mainland), surf pictures on the walls, a new surfboard to ride, and even a surf adventure. Yep, right there on Waikiki beach, August 18, we sat on the fringe of a baptism luncheon held by our church. We solemnly watched the baptismal service, trying to feel joy for others, although pain was the only emotion surfacing for us.

Brother was extremely anxious about eating in front of other people; acknowledging this feeling, I gave him the option of eating in the car in private or finding a secluded space on the beach. He struggled to decide and seemed to want to answer what he felt was "right"—attending the baptism—yet he was visibly shaken by the thought of eating in front of other people. So I made an executive decision to spread a blanket next to a tree, approximately twenty feet away from the crowd, and we turned our backs to them, allowing some privacy for his eating but conceding to his obligatory side.

It was hard just being there. His friends from before his summer away wanted to be near him and talk to him and catch up—yet he literally could not handle this. He was aloof and constantly moving his legs or body in palpable anxiety and distress. He avoided eye contact and stayed near me. In his internal discomfort, several times his eye grew large in panic as tears flowed, and he began squeezing the food as if to crumble it and discard it. My gently placing a hand on his arm and consoling him helped us to work through many such moments until the meal could be finished.

When that obligation had passed, he begged to get in the water and permission was granted under the watchful eye of Angel Kirsten, who attends our church and volunteered to go with him. It was his first opportunity to get in the water since our return home. They paddled out on her stand-up paddleboard and joined some of the other church and family members in the water. A short time later, they paddled back in, or should I say, Angel Kirsten paddled Brother back, reporting that he had tried to lift himself on a surfboard, but he had been shivering uncontrollably and unable to exert even enough energy to lift his small frame onto the piece of fiberglass. He would have never made it back to shore without her assistance. Terrorist Joey had taken from Brother the very thing he most wanted! I was upset by this reality and retrieved my child, warming him with a towel, only to realize even that was insufficient to mitigate his shivering. He bristled under my touch.

No activity was normal anymore. We could not be around other people in any social setting because people would make Brother agitated. We couldn't be anywhere food was present without a visible reaction in my child. And now I realized he had no strength or energy to participate in the smallest of playful moments.

The health complications this weakness represented were dire. According to Dr. Le Grange, a prominent specialist in the field: "If weight loss is not reversed, major medical complications, such as bradycardia, peripheral edema, and osteoporosis, may develop. Numerous other complications can also result from AN: interference with physical development, growth, and fertility, generalized and occasional regional atrophy of the brain, poor social functioning, low self-esteem, and high rates of comorbid substance abuse, mood disorders, anxiety disorders, and personality disorders." (5) Part of that medical risk, according to Dr. Erik Ulland, is that "during teen to late twenties, the brain is myelinating itself, which basically involves wrapping longer pathways in fat for insulation for faster signals. It is this process that allows thirty year olds better ability to stop impulses. Or thirty to fifty year olds better ability to process larger amounts of information than a younger brain." Therefore, fat is a necessary component for brain development! Terrorist Joey does not disclose this to his victims.

Brother's follow up medical appointment was telling. The pediatrician who examined him at Hickam Air Force Base had received Brother's inpatient report, and out of concern, she ordered a battery of tests. He had another EKG that, thankfully, was normal.

His blood pressure showed signs of malnourishment, and he was extremely constipated, backed up clear through his colon. In addition, he was borderline anemic and his white blood cells were abnormal. His iron levels were low and he had lost some basic reflexes. Sitting on the examination table with the doctor, puzzled as to why his knee did not respond to the metal hammer, was a strange phenomenon for the doctor and me. Brother's mental state, however, rendered him oblivious.

Psychologically, Brother was overly conscious about his midsection and unable to allow the doctor to examine him without tears and intense anxiety and stiffness. Her concerns were amplified enough to send him to a military adolescent medical doctor who would have more experience with this illness. We went there and were referred one more time to a community-based medical professional who was able to claim specialty status with this complex disorder.

This doctor was thorough and patient with us. She confirmed that his blood pressure was affected by the lack of nutrition as evident in her examination. She worried about his growth having been stunted. In addition, she explained to me that in the course of her physical exam, she noticed he had developed lanugo on his back. Lanugo is the fine white hair that covers a fetus in the womb; it sometimes remains when a baby is born because of its tiny frame and need for body warmth. Other than being a characteristic of the newborn, lanugo's appearance is a rare phenomenon that is only seen in severe weight loss cases of anorexia. (6) His body had reverted to infant-like measures to preserve life! This was shocking to hear and news to me since he would not allow me to see him uncovered to any degree. Her recommendation was to continue his meal plan and eating regimen combined with psychiatric and nutritional support and return for a follow-up examination soon. This multidisciplinary help had already been arranged and initiated; therefore, we continued straddling all three professions in a desperate attempt to stabilize Brother's condition.

Tripler Army Medical Center is a pink brick hospital on a historic hill, named Red Hill, in the heart of Honolulu. Red Hill is where, since World War II, the United States Armed Forces have stored the Pacific Fleet fuel supply to prevent catastrophic endings to attacks such as Pearl Harbor and preserve the potential war saving resource—*fuel*. See, even a country needs fuel to survive.

It was a symbolic location for our own personal battle. It was here that Brother and I first met with a psychiatrist on-island and reviewed the current symptoms and eating challenges. The psychiatrist asked a lot of questions, and I provided as many answers as I could, although my own questions outnumbered his.

Brother sat there numbly on the edge of his seat, his face filled with anxiety, until the dam burst and he began crying, unable to speak. That was all he could do. I was told we needed to meet weekly and would be working with the doctor's supervised resident. I objected moderately inside and meekly outwardly, requesting my son work with the male psychiatrist himself, whom I had sought out to provide a same gender perspective and who had a positive reputation as a more seasoned doctor. However, I was reassured that Brother would get optimal care from the doctor assigned, so I complied.

I had done extensive research and asked around the medical community to ascertain the best fit for my child, and because I am in the field of mental health, I am more than aware that not all framed degrees on the wall are alike. I wanted the best. I needed the best. Brother was more than a statistic to me. He was my flesh and blood and one of the two reasons I believe I was put on this planet.

We went twice. The therapist was a kind and empathic woman who listened to my concerns, asked me to step out of the room, and allowed Brother time to share what he could. She weighed my child on a scale and then set up a follow-up session. She was caring and genuine, and for that, I am grateful.

What I was unprepared for in my hyper-vigilance against anything that started with the letter "p" (purging) was for session two to start with an explanation of how laxatives can help with stomach pain connected to constipation. "It's a fine white powder that doesn't have any taste and tastes pretty good with milk," the therapist explained to my vulnerable and susceptible child.

What? My mind started reeling. I wanted to plug Brother's ears and erase what he had just heard. He doesn't need to know another way to rid his body of calories!

It was well-intentioned advice but potentially deadly. All the while, I had been secretly drugging him on the advice and prescription of his medical doctor with a powdered laxative to help his body process the newly introduced foods. I just happened to believe he was on a *need to know* basis, and he did not need to know this. I forced a smile and said, "Thank you very much." We walked out that day, and I knew we would not be back. Brother melted down in the parking lot, convinced his shadow was evidence of his fatness.

> ***TIP #5:*** *Anorexia is a fragile medical condition. Handle it with care, utmost vigilance, and be the gatekeeper against binging and purging opportunities. Never allow access to either opportunity if at all possible.*

When my heart is overwhelmed,
lead me to the rock that is higher than I.

– Psalm 61:2

CHAPTER 6

OUR NEW NORMAL

The first four months of Brother's treatment were a complete haze—a haze of doctor appointments, nutrition appointments, psychiatric appointments, group meals, grocery store runs, meltdown management, researching this illness and how to treat it, and communicating between all primary players. Life as we knew it before had ceased. Our new normal was cumbersome.

Although she steered us in the right direction through referrals and recommendations, Angel Ingrid had offered to be my friend, rather than Brother's counselor. She provided a supportive role rather than a professional one. After a great deal of runaround and referral chasing the first week on the island, I had chosen to work with a nutritionist in the community who came highly recommended. She worked as a team with a psychiatrist who agreed to provide the therapy component. It was an exclusive arrangement, and I was told I could work with both or neither—I chose both. This phone consult helped solidify my decision for where to take Brother for psychiatric help. The nutritionist provided individual consultation and meal planning, group meals twice weekly for eating disordered clients, and also ran a support group for parents and families.

The feeding group consisted of some recovered sufferers and some children/adolescents in all stages of treatment. Brother went every Tuesday and Thursday evening after school to help normalize eating with positive peer support and to help develop accountability for eating outside the home environment. Since mealtime was a power struggle six times a day this group was valuable backup for me and reinforced with my son that he was no longer going to be allowed to self-starve. Some things are negotiable in life as a child; eating was not!

Between the nutritionist and psychiatrist, their dual treatment process was broken down to me in terms of three stages: (1) weight restoration, (2) challenging distorted self-image, and (3) exploring family dynamics underlying this dysfunction. This was an adapted approach that incorporated some Maudsley methods with conventional family structure exploration. The strictly Maudsley approach follows the first two phases with less emphasis on family systems and more on adolescent identity formation in the third stage.

Renowned Maudsley experts Daniel Le Grange, Ph.D. and James

Lock, MD, Ph.D., break the stages into (1) weight restoration, (2) giving food control back to the teen, and (3) development of healthy identity formation.(5)

There is a great deal of overlap in these treatment methodologies, which place emphasis in slightly different camps. According to both strict Maudsley protocol, as well as that of our treatment team, we were in phase one. For my son, this weight restoration ended up taking approximately ten weeks. For some patients, it never ends.

During this time, Brother's diet consisted of high calorie foods and powerful nutritional supplements. He remained at a 3,500 calorie per day intake goal. This smelt like thick bacon cuts in the morning and looked like a slice of pie to wash down his whole milk, with whipped topping as a bonus.

Brother protested, claiming I was just trying to make him fat. Somehow, his definition of fat had gotten off track. Truly, I was trying to fatten him up—in the sense of having body mass that would cover the protruding bones! Not the definition of fat that means overweight. But he was unconvinced.

With some meals, he would go along as expected; at other times, he would bargain and try subversive measures to avoid ingestion. One day, I recall finding food remnants in the folds of the couch, but most of the time, he would passively try to leave behind small bites of food on his plate or on the floor and just avoid total consumption.

At school, he would try tactics such as "accidentally" spilling his juice or dropping food on the ground, rendering it inedible. I pictured Terrorist Joey with a stake in the ground, trying to say, "Oh, yeah, take that." This is why Brother needed to be watched at all times. He only ate because he now had no choice. He only drank because he was required to.

I felt immense pressure to make sure he gained weight rapidly because the professionals explained it was one of the primary indicators of a good prognosis...and I was desperate for that. As desperate, I imagine, as a mother who sees her child being abducted in front of her eyes, or as a father watching his child die from organ failure when all he needs is a donor transplant. It was a desperation that is hard to convey in words, but it was tangible to me. I could taste it, sense it, feel it, and breathe it. Every meal was a fight not to slip over the edge. Every grocery store trip became as important as a medevac operation to deliver a needed organ.

My peripheral vision had disappeared at the moment of our reunion and all I could see from that day on was this mission. Its heaviness was amplified by the professionals repeating over and over that the person most responsible for implementing their suggestions was me. The one most capable of intervening was me. And the one most tasked with project Heal Brother was me.

Overthrowing the villain was a full-time job. Yet I was greatly empowered by my authority as a parent, my privilege to decide when he could not decide, act when he could not act, and think when he could not think. Upholding me through it all was the God of the universe who decided in His unfathomable wisdom that this was *adversity with meaning* and a refining time in my child's life as well as my own. I remember thanking God continuously that my child was going through this at thirteen and not twenty-one. I still had the power that came with his living under my roof and monitoring eyes!

My heart stuck in my throat as I sat in the eating disorder group, listening to a thirty-something-year-old woman share how this illness had robbed her of two decades of life. It had robbed her of a normal adolescence where you go to parties and movies and don't avoid social places because food is involved. It robbed her of the mental and physical health required to obtain a college education. It robbed her of financial independence, and it robbed her of motherhood because she was too sick to care for her own child when he entered the scene. She had little to no recollection of the first years of her son's life because she was so weak she had to pass his care on to family members. And she lived with horrible regret and sadness over what Terrorist Joey had taken from her. Her terrorist might have been named Anna or Mia or Veronica. It was the same result, a room full of children and adults who had been misled and convinced of their "unworthiness" and felt their self-worth was conditional upon their body size.

In the craze of all that had taken place, I began to realize that Brother was losing out on life as well. He had no social awareness, was unable to hold more than a brief conversation, disliked normal activities of interest, had no stamina, was on an exercise ban medically, had no concentration for homework, and was failing all his classes and likely to be forced to repeat the eighth grade. I felt a surge of anger that the thing that didn't matter (waist size) was taking over things that did matter (living).

My agenda became clear—to help my son win the battle with minimal life experience casualties. When Brother wanted to surf, I wanted him to be capable of surfing. When he felt like spending time with friends, I wanted him to be social and able to connect with peers. When he was ready to date, I wanted him to date. When he was ready to play baseball, I wanted to cheer him on. When he felt like laughing at a joke, I wanted to laugh with him. All of this came to a screeching halt for him when he became ill.

Every week, I pulled him out of school at least twice for therapy and nutrition appointments. Once more for medical appointments as needed. This meant he was missing a great deal of school. He also would be pulled out of class for his morning monitored snack, and since this took forty-five minutes to an hour on average, he would miss more than an entire class period. In addition, his lunch period was extended due to the amount of time it took him to eat his lunch in entirety...two-three hours typically. In total, a lot of academic time was missed.

I tried hard to accept that life had to be this way right now. We quickly developed a chaotic routine that involved a day appointment with Brother's nutritionist weekly and two evening group sessions. He hated going to these appointments. The dietician was a very stern woman who directly stated she "played the heavy" for the parents. She was the authoritarian in this battle against self-starvation and she didn't mince words. She told it like it was, and she called him out on his anorexic behaviors.

Our visits always started with a blind weigh in. She would open the door and sometimes smile, sometimes not, usually with a look that suggested "Whatcha been up to?" with slanted brows toward Brother. *Convince me you are following the regimen* was the unspoken message. She then asked him to remove his sweatshirt, which by itself was enough to make him dislike her. She would calculate his weight and would report it to me without his awareness, sometimes in a whisper—other times written on a sticky note. It was secretive business. We couldn't let Terrorist Joey know the scale score.

It was important that Brother not fixate on a number because no *number* was ever going to be okay in his mind. He felt fat even as his organs were decomposing, so numbers were irrelevant!

After accomplishing this first and foremost matter of business, the dietician would alternate between speaking with me privately and him individually and sometimes us together as a family. The agenda of these sit downs was to assess how he was eating, observe him eat, look for problem behaviors, and talk with him about the anorexic life...what he was doing, what he needed to be doing, and how to fight this unseen monster. She wasn't the encouraging type, yet she knew this illness.

She would eat with him when these sessions could be timed during his lunch or snack. Sometimes, this eating occurred in public restaurants but primarily in the privacy of her office. The group meals alternated between catered in and eating out experiences. She was extremely helpful in educating me about this disorder, what to expect, and ways to counteract Terrorist Joey's tactics. A rule of thumb that helped immensely was to understand: *There is no bad food*. One symptom of eating disorders is to classify certain foods as allowable and others as taboo. That may sound pretty common and normal; however, the problem with this labeling is that unlike a healthy brain, the disordered brain continues to add to the "taboo" list and shrink the "acceptable" list.

She gave practical suggestions for how to manage Brother's odd behaviors, including numerous obsessions and compulsions that complicated his illness.

The psychiatrist was a direct contrast in terms of personality. Empathetic and with smiles that seemed easy to give, she took a therapeutic approach to treating Brother. She asked for family history and symptom evolution and lent a listening ear. Ever since the experience with the *laxative therapist* our first week back on island, we had maintained a bi-weekly regimen with the dietician and psychiatrist team. This dual approach seemed efficient, effective, and expedient. Which translated to...feasible, in single parent language. I mentally leaned into the idea that my son was working with the best providers and was receiving the best care possible.

> ***TIP #6:*** *Blind weigh-ins are important. Avoid the scale and measuring tape unless used by a health professional and keep the information away from the child. Do not allow the child to fixate on a number or other comparative means. Prevent this as much as possible.*

Mental anguish always results from
the avoidance of legitimate suffering.

— Stefan Molyneux

CHAPTER 7

TERRORIST JOEY

I hesitate to introduce you to Terrorist Joey. But I promised...so I will. To understand Brother's journey you have to understand his attacker. However, it seems to me that an introduction to someone or something should be done under good terms. Yet here I sit and type, and as the cursor moves across the page and those letters spill out, my blood boils.

I hate Terrorist Joey.

"Hate" is strong language, but honestly, it is not strong enough. Scratch that.

I despise Terrorist Joey. I loathe him.

He is an essence, a presence, a persona, a mind game—conceptually a strange concoction of brain chemicals, subconscious forces, spiritual influence, damaging family dynamics, and thinking gone awry. Somewhere between the spaces of the cerebral cortex with live wires, chemical input, hormonal surge, and neurotransmitter signals, a cavity was invaded and this poison spread until the damage was evident in every aspect of this young boy's existence.

When I use the term poison, I don't mean it literally, but it had the same pervasive and destructive effect over his life. Terrorist Joey convinced Brother to starve. No, he demanded Brother starve, and in exchange, he promised wonderful things would come. Brother's starvation turned into a physical nightmare that was equivalent to running a train off track and down a steep ravine—with equal momentum. There was no going back without food nourishment at a cellular level. And Terrorist Joey had cut off that supply.

You may wonder where such a villain gets the name Joey. You see, in my research, I had come to learn that the first recourse in reclaiming one's mind from anorexia is to realize that the thoughts regarding body image and starvation come from outside of oneself. In other, somewhat clinical terms, one has to *externalize* the illness. The person is not the illness. Just as someone with leukemia is not cancer. And someone with MS (multiple sclerosis) is not MS. Rather *Sally who has cancer,* or *Joe who has multiple sclerosis*. Therefore, my child was not Brother *the* anorexic. He was Brother *with* anorexia. And the goal was to eradicate the *with*.

The mental state I had to come to was full awareness that my son was not the impetus behind the food restriction; he was not the source behind the anxiety; he was not the thought behind the pacing.

He had been hijacked.

Knowledge is power, and this momma needed power. As I realized the importance of separating the child from the mental torturer, I intentionally used this differentiation in my talks with my child. I would say, "I am raising you, Brother, not Anorexia. Anorexia can get out of my house." My phraseology included, "Let me talk to Anorexia right now," and "I know this is hard for you, Brother, and that voice inside your head is loud, but please ignore it and trust mine."

I used the analogy with Brother that when he was young, he trusted my voice to tell him when to get out of the street or distrust strangers. Now the danger was just as real, so he needed to trust my voice and ignore the luring predator in his head. When I broke it down this way, he would look at me with the innocence of a toddler and briefly nod or give body language indicative of his considering it.

I am convinced that Brother struggled to distinguish these thoughts himself and needed a trusted adult to do it for him—to pull him out of the mental quicksand in which he was drowning.

Brother's psychiatrist was hugely instrumental in this mental fight.

She broke everything down simply. Therapist-assigned homework, session one: Give that voice in your head a name. Struggling with my own desperation, I was not about to let this homework assignment slide! So, I had a conversation with Brother that night... "What should we name it?" He shrugged and tried to change the topic. I persisted and he laughed while looking directly at me and said with strange sincerity, "Joey, since he is my best friend."

He was serious. I'll be! No thank you. This *thing* that had thrust itself into our life uninvited...a *friend*. I wanted to crawl out of my skin. Swallowing hard, I conceded some middle ground, thus the pseudonym Terrorist Joey came to be. Aka Liar. Destroyer. Hijacker. Life Killer. I could go on and on. But at least we now had language for *it*. Language to separate *it* from *him*, the one I love.

His nightly prayer illustrated greatly his lack of insight into his presumed friend *Joey*, yet it also spoke about his great need and subconscious plea for help:

"Dear Jesus, Please help the kids who are starving in Africa."

End prayer. This was it. Simple. Powerful. And strikingly ironic. This is the prayer my emaciated son prayed nightly during his first few months back in my care.

He could barely hold a conversation and said very little in the way of normal give-and-take dialogue. This was the case even in his supplication toward the God he loves. However, he did send this one petition to the throne room: Help the starving children.

How could he not see that he was that starving child! Most likely he knew deep down. He knew he needed help, but since he could not help himself and could not admit he needed to eat, this prayer was the closest his psyche got to asking. The mind is a fascinating and complex organ. His prayer was a projection of his heart's cry. My ears were listening. My heart was aching. And God was working.

> ***TIP #7:*** *Externalize the illness. Your child is not anorexia. Your child HAS anorexia nervosa or bulimia nervosa or another form of eating disorder not specified. Your child IS Brother, or Sally, or Steven, or Molly. Focus on supporting the child you know and combating the invader.*

The sorrow which has no vent in tears
may make other organs weep.

— Henry Maudsley

CHAPTER 8

A BLOODY REALITY

He had a bloody stool and cried out in fear. "Mom, come here!" There was a substantial amount of blood in the toilet. As if my pubertal teen had started her period, but I don't have a daughter, I have a son. This wasn't normal.

I called the doctor and explained what I had seen. My fear that it was abnormal was confirmed. But we could do little except wait and see whether it happened again. In my sleep-deprived state, I neglected to obtain a stool sample; determined not to do that again, I armed myself with plastic gloves, a stool sample cup, and a plastic Ziploc bag *in case*. If it happened again, Brother would have to see a gastro-intestinal specialist to rule out further complications, and I wanted to provide materials to solve this mystery. A new rule emerged in our household—no flushing. We regressed to prehistoric days. No flushing meant no vomit went down the drain, no bloody stools unnoticed, and no opportunity for Terrorist Joey to convince Brother that "No one will know" if calories disappeared down the white porcelain bowl. So we existed like this for a while.

Other accommodations were made also. Such as no doors locked. And I even contemplated taking the door off the hinge after I heard another parent recommend it in the support group we attended. Apparently, although rare, Brother was not the only male child in our civilized society trying to control tough emotions through self-starvation. But it was much more common among teen girls and, sadly, they were present in the support group also.

This family support group was where I came face-to-face with other hurting and confused parents and children. I ate up the group minutes like a starved parent, starved for help, frantic for answers, desperate for solutions. In the business district of Honolulu, one Monday a month, crowded into a meeting room, were approximately twenty-five sets of parents. When I scanned the room, my heart sunk upon realizing I was the lone single parent there.

Self-doubt crept in.

What was I up against? Again, *could I* do this?

Next to these stressed out faces were varying ranges of emaciated and even full-bodied forms—some subtle, some obvious, and some secretive. All of them were severely hurting internally.

I distinctly recall our first meeting. Brother sat on the very edge of his seat, moving his legs anxiously, and he seemed unable to sit back or sit still. His mouth clenched tightly and then released, only to tighten again and release, and his hands grasped his stomach region or locked around his thighs subconsciously. His demeanor matched that of many other frightened looking children. He was suspicious and wary of the group's intentions...to take away his control over food. No way! Force me to eat. Scary! It was as if Terrorist Joey and Brother were wrestling inside, and the victor was yet to be determined.

I listened aptly and took mental notes. "Cover mirrors," they said. Cover mirrors I did. That night even. No room for error or delay here. Immediately following the meeting, we went to a local store and hunted for paper blinds to cover every mirror in our home with the exception of my room. Amazingly, it helped avoid some emotional meltdowns. When Brother couldn't *see* himself, he couldn't *perceive* wrong, at least visually. This was only a short reprieve, though, because he would feel his body and panic or see himself in everyday household objects, which would trigger him. He saw his reflection in my coffee maker so that had to be covered. And the microwave, and the front hallway window to the outside world. Even his deodorant bottle was a reflective object and caused an anxiety spell on numerous occasions. I banned use of sunglasses in our family because they would set him off. All of these served as reflective devices, and the image he saw was clearly not the image the world saw.

Our whole daily routine shifted because of this invader. One evening, out of desperation and need for a projective tool, I asked Brother to draw a body outline. Here is what he drew: ("Giggles" is a misspelled "Jiggles." More evidence of his cognitive deterioration since spelling was one of his strengths and he had taken second place in his fourth grade spelling bee.)

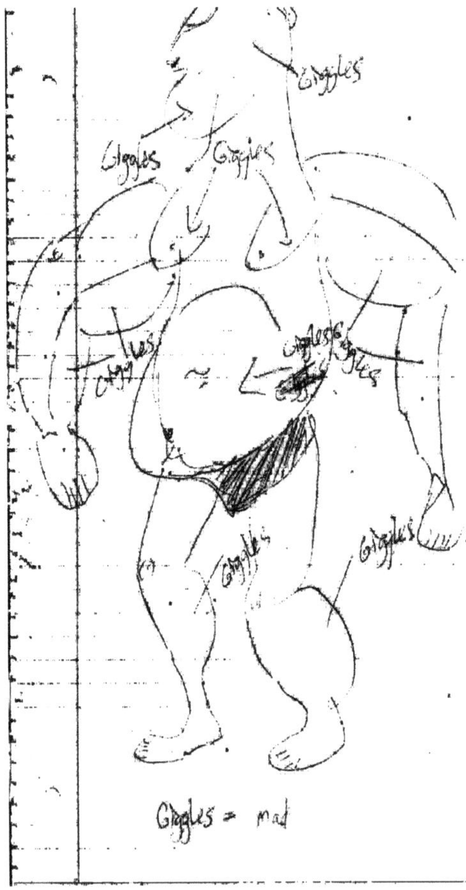

Immediately after drawing the first image, he asked for another piece of paper. Here is what he drew:

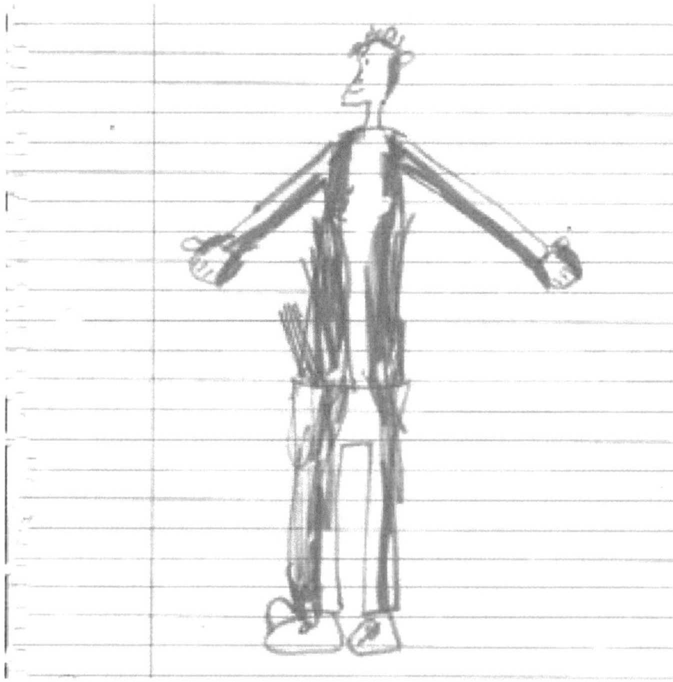

Then he made sure he clarified to me that it was "only the non-shaded parts, Mom." The shaded parts, he said, were a mistake. With horror, I noted that the clear space is what he looked like in the hospital! I have some training with child therapy art techniques, and what I noticed was the gigantic image had no facial features and lacked a head of hair. It had no expression and was distorted in form and size. The stick figure drawing had facial features and depicted an inverted face. It also possessed a full head of curly locks, which he identified with, and sported his school uniform (school initials whited out for this printing). My personal interpretation was that Brother identified with the second, smaller image and wanted to be such, while he was trapped feeling like the first one. He was a spitting image of the stick figure, minus the inverted face and sans the smile.

Until anorexia nervosa showed up on my doorstop, I remember thinking with disbelief, "Surely, these people do not think they are fat when they look in the mirror! Impossible. They are walking skeletons!" It is hard to comprehend because the healthy brain has no template for this. Only after walking through the pit of this mind game with my son has my understanding shifted to one of sad realization—perceiving and feeling *fat* while *thin*—is indeed their reality. Anorexia (AN) is truly a disorder of the mind. Before AN, Brother saw a normal reflection. During AN, he saw fat, and only fat. And after healing, a normal perception is amazingly restored.

TIP #8: *The ill child does not see what we see. Anorexia is a disorder of the mind and heavily influenced by cognitive errors and distorted thinking and perception. Cover the mirrors and take away reflective objects or cover them. Do this in the child's room as well as shared living spaces. Avoid reflective objects as much as possible in public places. Minimize opportunities for the brain to be tricked.*

Pets are humanizing.
They remind us we have an obligation and
responsibility to preserve and nurture
and care for all life.

— James Cromwell

CHAPTER 9

THERAPEUTIC PAWS

Pets. Furry animals, hairless ones, ones that bark, meow, hop, crawl, and even swim. Companions. Needy. Dependent on the hand that feeds them. They eat, drink, and poop. Everything that eats goes through this predictable cycle. When I was reunited with my son in late July, clearly he was not doing the former—I am not sure he was doing the latter. He rarely used the restroom and medically was very *backed up* since the food transportation highway had shut down unexpectedly. Animals were an acceptable route to reconnect him with this cycle.

Historically, my son had a big heart for animals of all kinds. He seemed to understand their legitimate need for food and liquid. Angel Ingrid suggested I take Brother to the Humane Society so we would become volunteers.

That is exactly what we did. The three of us in our bedraggled family put on our long pants, tennis shoes, and joined the volunteer orientation class in the hopes of getting access to the green apron that would perhaps pull on the heart strings of this starved mind.

Domesticated animals are dependent on humans for care and sustenance. The animals at Hawaii Humane Society became secret recruits for Project Heal Brother. To care for others mirrors the need to care for oneself, and Brother continued to feel compassion for others. He had just shut down responding to his own needs.

One sunny Saturday morning, we followed the directions to the prearranged classroom and met with the director and her staff along with numerous other compassionate souls. We listened to the schedule of care these animals required on a daily basis and learned how to be part of that team. We toured the facilities and were briefed on how to hold, play with, and love on a variety of species, including rats! Shiver. We were then issued those fabulous green aprons and given key access.

I looked at my children with anticipation and asked them one question, "When do you want to start?" "Now! Please, Mom!" said my younger child, who was eager and giddy with excitement. Brother seemed ambivalent and unreachable, which was abnormal and dramatically different than his unhijacked self. So I decided there was no time like the present.

But first, a snack for my own young was in order! I grabbed the bag of goodies I had brought along and walked with the kids to a nearby park. My youngest child and I sat down...normally. Brother sat on the edge of the bench as if he wanted to lean into the wooden surface *just enough* to support his frame and *no more*. He appeared to be internally battling over how much space one's rear end actually needed to take up on a chair's surface! I handed him a bag of nuts, a power bar, and a juice. Each food item was prepackaged into a clear bag so no calorie references appeared on the packaging. I had caught him reading food labels, so I had devised this new trick to avoid another opportunity for Joey to mess with Brother. When I was not able to repackage, I would rip off labels or cross out caloric/fat gram information with a permanent marker.

Ha, Joey, I have powers of persuasion too! Brother was just given his bag with predetermined portions and a drink stripped of its label and expected to consume. Initially, he obeyed, but he began to struggle about halfway through.

"Why do I have to eat this much?" he complained. He stalled and bemoaned my excessive snack portions. With anorexia, any food is excessive, right? My task was to remain firm. "Eat before we go back," I demanded. "Or eat as we drive to the hospital. Or don't eat and the hospital staff will make sure you do. Your choice." This was my leverage and all I had. He begrudgingly and sloppily forced the rest of the food remnants down his throat and shed some tears as he complained about what a horrible mother I was. I'm pretty sure my breathing was slightly constricted every time food and Brother were in the same vicinity. Each eating encounter seemed like a mighty hill to climb, and each time we clawed our way to the top, I would subconsciously breathe out some audible relief. Whew.

"Okay, let's go back," I instructed. And we walked back. Well, younger son and I walked back. Brother zigzagged.

We went to the cat room first. I was secretly hoping to re-trigger Brother's interest in cats since we had owned two cats previously. They had been joy giving, loyal companions to this young boy at the time, but we had regretfully had to leave them with family on the mainland. Now, Brother acted as if he didn't care or even miss them. He seemed indifferent. So the experiment was to see how he acted around precious cats and kittens of all colors, ages, and stages.

We grabbed the key and entered the cat house. It was a small space, comparable to a small bathroom. A flicker of interest and a whole lot of anxiety and nervousness began radiating from Brother. We visited the adult cats, which had been separated based on vitality and ability to play well with others; they were deemed the healthier and more social of the lot. My youngest quickly found several cats to pet and dote on. I began petting one that was in my vicinity while I watched a cat come up to Brother and begin rubbing and purring affectionately at his leg.

When Brother caught my gaze, I read fear in his eyes. He was scared. Of what? Confidently, I prompted him to reciprocate the affection, yet he awkwardly held his arms at his side and seemed unsure of what to do. After several prompts and reassurance from me, he pet the cat briefly. He stood awkwardly in the corner as he did so while his younger brother and I had taken seats on the provided benches. I encouraged him to do the same, but he ignored me and remained standing.

After a while, we meandered through the door to an adjoined rectangular space with cages lined up alongside the wall. Several cats were separated into designated slots. Two other volunteers in the room had taken out one of the cats and were playing with her. The boys watched and Brother seemed transfixed. The cat was injured and vulnerable, and Brother watched with great interest. My youngest begged to take out another cat, but we took the advice of one of the volunteers to wait since that particular cat had some social anxiety and needed his space.

We spent some time with the other volunteers and then chose to enter the kitten section of the enclosed cat house. One might think that kittens are harmless and all children would relish the chance to cuddle with them. Every child there did...except Brother. He again stood awkwardly and remained distant. There were three small, white, fluffy kittens among a group of eight or so. A lively crew! They climbed the walls, pounced on toys, and hid behind boxes.

Lovingly and carefully, I picked up the white fur ball closest to me and began petting it. These kittens were pulling at my heart-strings. They were adorable!

I waited for Brother to reach out and pet one. He didn't. He stood as if he were trying to remain as far away from the kittens as possible. His eyes again met mine, this time with sadness and confusion evident in his enlarged irises. I whispered to him, "What is wrong?" He answered tearfully, "I will hurt them, Mom."

What! Are you kidding me? my mind screamed. Instead, my mouth was silent as I formulated a response. You see, I read body language for a living, so I had an advantage in analyzing this scene. He was terrified! Terrified that his emaciated body was too large to share this walk-in closet-sized area with these precious kittens. He believed himself to be giant, when in reality he was a stick figure. He refused to sit because he was afraid his body would crush the animals! He was afraid to bump into them because he feared he would hurt them! He was afraid to touch them, thinking it would do them harm.

Restraining the speech I wanted to give about how absurd his response was, I patted the bench with an encouraging nod. Sit down. It's okay. "Look at me," I said. "I am sitting and not hurting them. I am holding one and she likes it." After some convincing, Brother gingerly rested a quarter of his nearly nonexistent rear end on the bench and let the rest of his body hang out into space, as if to say,

"I don't want to be large enough to take up any space on this surface." He allowed the kittens to crawl over and around him, but he was unable to reciprocate the affection.

Out of respect for the growing crowd around the kittens, we moved on to the dogs. There were large and small breeds. Loud and quiet ones. I made an intentional comment as we walked past their cages about how great it was that there was such variety of animals and how we are all made with uniqueness and great care. Our bodies, like the animals, are meant to take up the space we do. Lots of different shapes. And it's okay. It's perfectly okay.

We gravitated toward a puppy that was barking and clamoring to be held. I grabbed a blanket to wrap him in, per society policy, and the three of us shared the burden of his energetic and muscular frame. This little guy was small, but powerful. Brother was loosening up just a bit and agreed to hold him, but not alone. Following his lead, we tackled this task as a team and then decided to call it a day.

This day at the Humane Society had been emotionally exhausting, but very informative. It held up a behavioral mirror to how much my son had lost—personality-wise, interactively, socially, as part of the world he belonged to. He was changed. And it made my heart sad.

Along with the idea to interact with feline friends, Angel Ingrid had given Brother a plant—a sunflower with wondrous growth potential, beautiful color and shape waiting to blossom. It was his—his alone to water and care for. He tackled this responsibility with devotion and seriousness. He regularly watered his plant. When he was tired, he watered this plant. When he was calm, he watered his sunflower. When he was angry or frustrated, he watered it still. It was more than a job. He cared! He wanted the flower to grow. He mentioned that it needed water and sunshine, so he positioned it by our front steps and by our outdoor sink, so it could have both readily. This sunflower appeared to open a portal into his old self. The old self that enjoyed life. Loved life. Here he was encouraging a life of some form. Even if it wasn't his life, it was symbolic and a connection to life in general.

It was troubling to observe the anorexic paradox—fixated on food and how much others need food, even plants, yet denying this need in his own existence! As an observer, I saw this illness as the ultimate act of self-loathing. Death by starvation. Not even a quick end to internal pain, but a slow and drawn-out suicide in which one shrinks away to nothing and rejects attempts to sustain life. Where did this self-loathing come from? Why did an amazing child, who outwardly appeared to have everything society says one needs, think himself unworthy of the space his body filled? I have my theories as his mother. I have my theories as a therapist. He didn't know his value and unconditional worth on this planet. He didn't grasp in his mind that regardless of his body, *he*, the soul of his person, was of infinite worth and irreplaceable. That it could be otherwise was inconceivable to me because I knew him. And loved him. And couldn't imagine a world without him.

Yet, he was not convinced. One day while he was watering his beloved plant, a gecko darted across our path. Brother looked at me and forlornly said, "I killed it, Mom."

"What?" I asked.

Brother fought back tears and looked away, ashamed, as he stammered out the sentence that he had tried to catch a gecko in our yard and had killed it, squeezing too hard in his eagerness. His words were harsh and self-condemning. He personalized this! Since he had been a young child of five or six, he had enjoyed catching those quick little ground hugging, scurrying lizards. He loved them. In fact, when we had lived in Germany for a couple of years, he had caught one to keep as a pet! He cared for it then and fed it flies, and he made sure it had the best ecology a boy could afford for his treasure!

With childish interest and gentle care, he tried to catch them without injury. I reminded him of this. *Keep talking son,* my mind whispered. *Let me hear your fears. They are illogical. They are untrue. They are distorted. They are planted there by the LIAR.* You see, he thought he had killed the gecko because he was "too fat." Strong equals too fat to the anorexic. Yet because he *knew* me...truly knew me and trusted me...he was slightly able to edge my truth into his brain full of lies and distorted reasoning as I explained that the gecko had not died because he, Brother, was too fat. Perhaps he had slightly miscalculated speed and force. Perhaps it had happened because the lizard was too quick and had moved too eagerly. His youthful hands had surely provided a safe cavity meant protectively to encapsulate his catch. He was a kid. Not a killer. Not a fat killer by any stretch of the imagination. If only Joey's imagination weren't so deviant! But during that conversation, I saw a small inch of his brain space reclaimed.

> ***TIP #9:*** *Provide opportunities for nurture and care of animals or plants if possible. Transfer this symbolism into messages and opportunities for the child's self-care. Simultaneously, avoid any exposure to packaging that displays caloric content or fat grams. This is irrelevant data and provides an opportunity for fixating on numbers—which is distortion fuel in the fragmented mind.*

We need to be tender and willing to show
compassion for others, but also have the strength
to confront situations that require resolute courage.

— Craig Williams

CHAPTER 10

TOUGH LOVE IS, WELL…TOUGH!

Things were escalating with Brother's eating. He took longer and longer to finish his meals and snacks, to the point that, despite being at school, he wasn't really at school. He was in the counselor's office getting one-on-one time eating each morsel with the pace of a turtle.

I think there are several plausible reasons for why this happened: First, getting fat was his greatest fear, and he was required to face bravely that fear six times a day. Therefore, the task of eating caused him a great deal of anxiety, so slowing down the food consumption was his mind's way of managing his nerves. A second factor was that since being reintroduced to foods, he outwardly objected to the nourishment because this disorder is one of only a few psychiatric illnesses that are *egosyntonic*, meaning the individual who has this condition does not want to change it because the restrictive behaviors are in line with his goals and values. (7) That person believes the food restriction is a means to an end—and refusing food will help him feel skinnier, which is connected in his fragmented mind to improved feelings of self-worth. Yet being truly hungry inwardly, when forced to consume, he must have savored each bite. His parent and the professionals required him to eat, so although accepting this was done with extreme internal conflict and distress, it was still food. And his body was hungry! This strange eating behavior was an outward expression of the tension in his inner world. He had an appetite and hunger pangs, but he felt like he was failing himself when he gave in to this basic primal need (keep in mind he had successfully controlled the urge to eat for nearly two months believing this restriction was the *right* thing to do to feel better about himself), and the voice in his head surely condemned him as he partook. Thirdly, he had compulsions to burn calories. As the calories went in, he had continuous urges to rid his body of those same calories. Chewing for extended periods of time was a passive aggressive way of fighting the requirement to eat—and in his mind—getting fat.

With all of this storm inside, his eating became more and more unmanageable, and our time was less and less our own. Terrorist Joey likes to monopolize that as well. Ensure, that six-pack, was called into duty. His nutritionist instructed me to give him one bottle if he was not able to complete his meal in a forty-five minute time frame. Two bottles if he refused an entire meal. This expectation seemed impossible because his eating had been extended to two to three hours on average—each time! We had to shift this three-hour marathon into a forty-five minute timeframe, but how? Yet we could not go on with our mornings, afternoons, and evenings dictated by the eating process. Brother was informed of this and was given ample reminders. He would say that his stomach hurt and grasp his midsection. He would complain and stall. I watched the clock: Forty. Forty-one. Forty-two. Forty-three. Forty-four. Forty-five. Groan. This meant I had to give him Ensure, and that was the last thing I wanted. I wanted him to eat the food, real body nourishing morsels, and I honestly didn't want to enforce this expectation, knowing that a full-out battle would ensue. When I gave him the can anyway, he looked at me with fury and screamed and shook the bottle, pouring out its contents onto the table.

I cleaned up the table, trying to remain calm, and reached into the fridge for a second can. This was placed in front of him. He visibly started to shake and rage and grabbed the can to throw it. I stabilized the can, put the cap on, and firmly told Brother he had to drink one without destroying it or I would up the ante to two.

He drank it, tearfully, and with hurtful language. He yelled over and over again, "I hate you! You are the devil! I hate you!

I responded, "I love you," and "I know this is hard."

And he would storm away to scream and yell for minutes on end.

His tantrums were consuming. Sobs would wrack his body, and the volume of noise produced surely disturbed the neighborhood's peace. Sometimes, I would let it go on, but sometimes, I chose to intervene. I didn't know what to do most of the time and managed by trial and error. I wanted him to feel and be allowed to express the emotions he had internalized into this eating disorder, but he had to learn to manage these emotions in a healthy way. He had no such skills in this state.

The eating timeframe took about two weeks even to stabilize minimally. The threat of Ensure gave me leverage. He would always receive a timed warning and numerous reminders before the Ensure would be given. But it was a recourse used both at home and at Angel Kirsten's. She called me a couple of times, explaining Brother was sitting at her countertop, refusing his afterschool snack and getting irate when she proceeded to give him the liquid nutrition. Epic power struggle. I got on the phone with him and explained he would drink *one* for her or *two* for me, and I would come directly from work if I needed to.

And I meant it. I dropped everything when needed to enforce this expectation. He had to know beyond a shadow of doubt there was no option or he would have given in to the terrorist inside!

He drank and he screamed and he cried and he lashed out—even physically. During this time, we had some serious encounters that seemed possession like. Some days I questioned my safety as well as that of my youngest child. Yet it was clearly not my oldest son who hated me. I knew that to my core. It was the persona, the voice, the thought changer, the evil one.

As Brother's eating patterns became better, his moods became worse. I became the target of his anger as did his other caretakers. We were, after-all, the ones feeding him, so it made sense for Terrorist Joey to lash out and want to fight hard.

With persistence and consistency, the Ensure consequence seemed to work on the food timing issue, and eventually, we came to meet the forty-five minute expectation. Then, at some point, his nutritionist and psychiatrist suggested Ensure be used to change his obsessions and compulsions also. His malnourished brain had developed odd walking patterns, counting behaviors, sitting postures, body checking, etc. that were increasing and monopolizing his functioning.

Of all the OCD behaviors that escalated, the most noticeable and targeted was Brother's pacing. He *only* stood or paced. Never sat. The incessant nature of this behavior was termed "excessive movement" by his treatment team, and it was heavily discouraged. Apparently, it is a common symptom in the eating disorder world. Common for a child (or adult for that matter) to develop obsessive and compulsive mannerisms and to exert unnecessary energy. The behaviors were likely calorie-burning in his mind and passive-aggressive attempts to fight the weight gain phase. Even when walking somewhere, he would take the longest route possible.

One place this behavior was constantly evident was walking to the car. Our home had a side entrance and driveway directly to the right of the house when standing inside, facing the street. Brother would walk out the door, do an abrupt left, then walk straight, parallel with the vehicle, until he was behind the parked SUV, and then he would walk the long way around the vehicle from the left side to take a seat in the rear, right passenger side. A functioning brain takes a direct route to a destination...which would have been perpendicular to the vehicle and straight left to the parked vehicle. One mid-September evening, I decided I had to follow through with the Ensure consequence to stop this walking trajectory. I had given Brother verbal warning and, although he would stop the movements when directed, he would just restart immediately after with the same or a different compulsive movement, all of them energy-burning and excessive. We needed to head to evening meal time with his nutritionist and peer eating group, but he intentionally walked the long route around the car and made these unnecessary calorie burning movements. I produced an Ensure from my purse, my latest accessory, and required that he drink it. He screamed, flailed his arms, threw the liquid contents across the front seat, pleaded, and begged—all because of a bottled drink. This was dramatic, extreme, and unnecessary for a reasonable, healthy brain!

Every parent knows when the tantrum starts that you can't reward the behavior; you have to enforce consequences if it is to stop. Even when it's hard—and *especially* when it's hard! I knew I would have to stand my ground and fight now or it would be a longer battle later. A longer battle later with anorexia could mean death! The stakes were high. I picked up the remnants of the first splattered bottle and then gave Brother another. He threw it again and wailed and screamed that he hated me and I was the devil. I handed him a third, leaving the cap on, and instructed him to take it off and drink when ready, and if he choose not to do so, he would be given a fourth.

He refused. I grabbed a fourth bottle. Two bottle casualties and two ready to enter the combat zone. He screamed horrible things and pleaded incessantly. He begged me not to make him drink it. "Please, PLEASE! MOM, PLEASE!" was shouted at me with a frightening intensity. I stepped out of liquid harm's way and expected compliance. I stood there with a stern parent face until both drinks were eventually drained. Brother and I were emotionally spent, yet it was time to go to group.

My youngest son came out of the house (I had instructed that he wait inside until the zone was safe) and climbed into the vehicle so we could leave. We drove to group; meanwhile, Brother continued crying and whimpering and breathing fast and hard.

We rode the elevator and walked into the meeting room. There, in front of teen girls, peer boys, and the nutritionist, Brother leaned over and vomited all over the carpet. It barely fazed him that there was an audience, and he continued crying louder and louder to the point where he seemed unable to catch a breath and appeared to be hyperventilating. Does this sound like a boy gaining social acceptance?

Clearly, the terrorist was a deceiver. So I steadied Brother, walked him to a nearby restroom, and coached him through deep breathing—in and out, in and out, count to five, slowly—saying silent prayers of thanks for my counselor training in my own mental space!

It took several minutes for him to try to follow my lead because it was complicated by a sneezing attack. Excessive sneezing. Something beyond anything he had done before or since. He sneezed over fifty times, and each one took away his ability to catch his breath.

I held his arms as he neared a complete panic state. We locked eyes and I breathed with him. Inhale slowly one, two, three, four, five. Exhale slowly, one, two, three, four, five. Inhale slowly, one, two, three, four, five. Exhale slowly, one, two, three, four, five. Over and over until he could regain some composure. He had spit up and drooled on his legs, arms, feet, and clothes. He didn't seem to care about the mess on him or around him. He was shaking and upset, yet he was able to rejoin the group and somehow managed to eat dinner that night.

The expectation from my end was that he eat dinner and understand that even this...tantrum...hyperventilating...episode...was not an *out*. Especially, it was not an out. Such would have reinforced the escapist behavior. The expectation from his nutritionist was that he clean his mess. She sent him home with the area rug he had vomited on and instructions to wash and return. This was a turning point. From that day forward, he stopped walking the long way around things and his pacing decreased significantly.

We talked when I picked him up later from the nutritionist run eating group. I explained that I hated knowing he had to go through that entire experience, and it made me immensely sad, yet I loved him enough to do it again. He nodded his understanding with a mixture of gratitude and respect shimmering in his eyes. The more I applied firm, tough love with care and empathy and compassion, the more he responded. His responses were validating and helped me down a path that felt mean, cruel, and demanding. I did the same when he was one and two and five and he needed structure to feel safe. I did the same during his early years when he needed immunization shots but screamed and fought back inconsolably. Now was no different, but the risks were higher in my mind. A parent doesn't ask a young child whether he want shots or not—a parent decides. Likewise, a parent doesn't ask a child with anorexia whether he wants to eat or not. The parent decides. Children can't see what is best for them; they don't have long-term perspective, and they can't evaluate consequences, especially in a mentally compromised state. This illness reminded me of the contrast between his youthful vulnerability and my parental obligation and privilege.

Because a child cannot understand long-term cause and effect until his or her brain has developed that cognitive skill and life experience has provided the raw data, a parent knows certain things to which the child is not privy. Terrorist Joeys capitalize on this vulnerability. My son did not know that depriving his body of adequate nutrition was destroying it, and at some unfortunate time during his food restrictive phase, he had succumbed to malnutrition and his brain had taken over. He was not in control of his decision making any longer. He had no mental awareness of the host of medical complications he was in danger of experiencing—one of them being a high risk for developing osteoporosis.

We had a talk one evening after he had been on the re-feeding regimen for some time. "Do you know what osteoporosis is?" I asked. "Osteo-what? No," he responded. I explained it was deterioration of bone structure and was a complication of anorexia. He looked shocked. And scared. Certainly not scared into eating. Nothing could do that. Yet this conversation put a seed of doubt in his head about the terrorist's lies.

This conversation was medically prompted. His posture had been reduced to that of a hunchback. He stooped over, unable or unwilling to extend his back fully. His doctor was concerned about scoliosis and recommended an x-ray to determine the level of curvature. I took him for such an exam, and the results were, thankfully, non-clinical, notwithstanding the technician's remarks, which were concerning: "Hmmm...strange, although there is only minimal signs of scoliosis and not to a harmful degree, his back is significantly curved in the image. Do you...think...he can control this or not?" she mused. Puzzled, I added to my list of things to accomplish that day: "Ask son if he can straighten back or not." Roger.

I felt like pinching myself to make sure I was still alert and oriented to reality. Nonetheless, I asked him and then watched as he struggled to sit up fully. He could straighten—sort of—but only when prompted and not easily. Clearly, over the course of the past few months, his body had adjusted to a stooped position that would take some conscious intention and time to re-straighten. From that day forward, I tried to remind him to stand *tall and proud*. When putting his dishes in the sink, I would come up behind him and say, "Tall and proud." Standing by the television, I would comment "Tall and proud." Walking to the car, I gave prompts of "Tall and proud." At times, these words helped him and he would stand just a bit more normally; other times, the words would cause a backlash of "Stop!" and "I know Mom," followed by tears. The anger roulette was worth it because momentum was building.

Tucking my children into bed used to be rather routine and simple. Talk about the day, pray, lean over, and kiss them—when they let me; they are boys after all! Tuck in the covers, literally on occasion, and say goodnight while turning off the light. For years, I had taken this simple gesture for granted. Now, Terrorist Joey stole this too. My son lay shivering under the blankets and layers of clothing and shied away from contact or touch. If I got within a twelve-inch radius of him, he would shrink away, avoiding touch or contact of any kind. If I sat too close or touched his skin, he would cry and moan, stating something about how fat he was...so fat there was no room for me even to sit on the bed.

I used to be able to sit on the edge of his bed and talk with him. No more. I compromised in this case. I kept my distance while we did our goodnight routine in a stifled manner, and then I came back for round two after he had fallen blissfully into the comfort of sleep and altered consciousness. Then I touched his hair, gently, but confidently. I prayed aloud, quoting Scripture. I refuted the evil influence that was badgering my son's mind, and I commanded it to leave. I claimed victory over this battle and pled with the God that gave this child breath to give him more time and a life free from anorexia.

It was during one of these moments, while touching his hair and praying, that I noticed with great sadness he didn't even sweat. Here he was in a very hot climate, in a room with no air conditioning, under a blanket and two layers of thick clothing, and not a drop of sweat was present. In contrast, I was in a tank top, shorts, and bearing a mixture of moisture from sweat and tears combined. How could this be? Dehydration was a reality, and the internal workings of his body were clearly still taking a hiatus. When you starve the body of basic nutrients and water long enough, the systems shut down and won't resume normal functioning immediately. It's like revving up an engine after a long, hard winter; the machinery doesn't remember what to do, how to work, or just plain doesn't have the juice it needs to function.

My nine-year-old son had requested a fan directly on him because it was so humid in the home. These were the hottest months in Hawaii. In contrast, Brother couldn't handle any breeze on his frail form, and in this physical state, he didn't sweat or seem bothered by the heat. It took nearly two months in this condition before I gratefully noticed beads of sweat around his head one evening. When that finally happened, thankfulness welled up in my throat. We were edging closer to victory. Winning meant living.

My youngest boy was complaining of a swollen finger joint and some other minor pains, so I made an appointment for him to see his primary care manager. It felt like we should pay rent at the doctor's office by now since it seemed to be a frequent destination for our struggling unit. I filled out the required paperwork and explained my concerns to the intake nurse. She had us follow her to a tiny cubicle, where, with the four of us crammed inside, my youngest was asked to step on the scale for a routine weigh-in and height check. Without hesitation, he did so as I non-verbally but directly, with laser eye glare (every mother knows the one!) motioned for my oldest to look away from the scale.

Brother was curious and wanted to know, I am sure, so he could compare and condemn himself for his own weight. He acted as if he wanted to be smaller than everyone...regardless of age. So here was this younger sibling four years his junior, and that was his competition for skinniest! It was all insane and surreal, but it was happening.

Brother was abnormally thin, skeletal at best. Here was my youngest...a *normal* child with a healthy body size and shape and zero concerns about his size. He was normal—whatever that meant. It was just, well, normal. And the digital number that came to my attention stopped my mind in its tracks. Seventy pounds. What? Seventy pounds!

The stark reality of the fact that here my youngest stood with his smiling, grinning, happy, jovial, eating self and at age nine weighed a healthy seventy pounds. The contrast hit me like a speeding train as I mentally computed the difference between the here and now weight of my youngest and the recent inpatient admittance weigh-in of my oldest...seventy-nine pounds. A measly nine pound difference.

My oldest had nearly wasted away a four-year growth period! His height told of his age, but his weight suggested major regression. The nurse ushered us into a nearby exam room and left us, saying the doctor would be with us soon.

My ability to stuff my own emotions was gone. I collapsed into the nearest chair, and holding my head in my hands, I sobbed.

Brother, now stiffly sitting on the edge of the seat next to me, subconsciously grabbed his stomach and whispered, "Mom, what's wrong?"

I glanced up and mumbled something to reassure him that I was okay.

But in reality, I wasn't.

> ***TIP #10:*** *Understand that obsessions and compulsions often coexist with eating disorders. These are attempts at controlling and dispensing of the extreme anxiety inside. And especially when the food control outlet is blocked, this transfers to other behaviors. Be a barrier to the expression of other dysfunctional obsessive and compulsive behaviors and rituals so they do not have a chance to become more entrenched. This is torturous (expect resistance)...but very important! You are the authority figure and the child desperately needs help regaining authority over his or her mind and behaviors. Do this ONLY with utmost love, compassion, patience, and empathy.*

We must face what we fear;
that is the case of the core of
the restoration of health.

— Max Lerner

CHAPTER 11

THE NEW "F" WORD

Fat was the three-letter F word. We avoided it and anything in its vicinity. Unless I was trying to figure out what was in Brother's head, which was my constant inquiry. Everyone was fat, it seemed. He believed his younger brother, age nine, was fat. He told me I was fat. My cousins and siblings called me "no butt" in high school because that was my skinny reputation. Now I know I am no longer a high school teen and most certainly have a fuller figure, but I don't believe fat would be a term used to describe me by anyone.

Yet my son believed in all sincerity that his whole healthy weight family was obese. He thought his friends were all fat, and every adult he crossed paths with was, in his evaluation, fat.

I wondered then, *What was skinny?* So I conducted a spontaneous research experiment one day in the car. As we were driving home,

I asked him as I pointed to innocent walkers and bikers and bystanders along our path, "Is he fat?" "Yes," he responded. "Is she fat?" "Yes." These poor people had no idea they were being evaluated and criticized by Terrorist Joey. One unsuspecting biker clearly had a six-pack and defined, muscular body, yet my son again responded with "Yes." I asked him then, "What is skinny?" He just shrugged like he had no idea.

Then an image of his emaciated body in the hospital crossed my cortex. I knew what he thought was thin, but it was deadly. His barometer was off! His ability to discern was compromised. And yet all he did on a continual basis was compare. Many days when I would pick him up after work from my friend's house, he would cry and bemoan that he was "fatter" than her daughters. Was this conversation really happening? Does a teen boy want to be skinner than the skinniest teen girls I knew?

Yep. My son did.

He seemed to hold it in until the privacy of our SUV afforded him the chance to release his tears and agony in this regard. He also hated his pictures, and the only image he moderately accepted at this point was on his school ID, taken less than a week after his release from the hospital. He had thrown away the first one, but come to a place of minimal acceptance of the second attempt. When he referred to this picture, he claimed it was better than older shots, although even it bothered him and seemed to display a *too fat* image for his distorted brain to accept.

I chose not to take pictures or visually document this time in his life. Photographs were too troubling to him, and there was no need to add to his discomfort. When he requested to opt out of the school yearbook, I agreed because it caused him pain, and to be honest, I wasn't sure I wanted to remember him this way.

Some previously normal activities were obviously a *no go* in our life now. We did not eat out at restaurants unless he was with his eating group because that involved an audience. We avoided the majority of social events. Sports and other after school activities were no longer on our to-do list. Our life consisted of managing grooming, work, school, eating, and moods.

Homework couldn't even make the short list. Literally, homework was a luxury I couldn't get to and Brother couldn't complete anyway, so we side-tabled it. When he did work on the occasional math problem, it boggled my mind how a gifted and talented math mind could struggle for thirty minutes to complete two basic math problems! Such is the demise of the mind without fuel.

As much as possible, I avoided stores and public places that had mirrors, food, people, or anything that might trigger an emotional episode for my son. Then one day I lapsed. Both of my sons needed a haircut, and although I usually cut their hair myself, I was extremely busy and tired and tried to downsize my list by one to-do item. We went to a local chain hairdresser shop and tried to fit in a quick cut. We discussed what Brother wanted, but as soon as he sat in the chair, my error registered: There were mirrors everywhere!

They were unavoidable. I thought about abruptly leaving, but Brother wanted this specific haircut and I was less than confident in my abilities at the moment due to how long his hair had become. We made eye contact and he fought back tears, but nodded his head affirmatively. So, following his lead, I calmly tried to communicate to the Asian hairdresser who spoke little English that my son had a medical condition that required we avoid mirrors, so please face him away from the main one and toward a wall instead. She struggled with this information and seemed not to comprehend. It was more than a language barrier, though; it was a strange request, so she just didn't get it.

Although the hairdresser initially faced Brother away from the mirror as requested, she kept talking to him about how he *surely* must want to see his cut, so she should turn him around. What wasn't directly said but implied was, *Your mom must be wrong; of course, you want to see!*

I wanted to scream and explain to this well-intentioned lady that she had no idea what we were dealing with. When she turned Brother around to face the mirror and continue her cut, I fought back my impulse to scream.

I sat on the edge of my seat, bouncing my leg like an anorexic patient myself, while hoping, praying, that Brother could manage this experience. He made it through the haircut but not without glances in the mirror toward my direction that clearly conveyed his distress. When his younger sibling took the seat for his turn, Brother came and sat by me, placed his hands in his lap, and just cried.

And it wasn't because of the cut. It was because of the reflection he saw. The hairdresser looked at me in surprise and I just nodded. *See. I tried to warn you!* I wanted to yell. But I knew it made no sense to the outside world because it made no sense to me. It made no sense to anyone. It was illogical and irrational. No-one would perceive this child as anything negative externally, yet that is all he could see for himself, and no outside influence could convince him otherwise. The world couldn't comprehend it or understand it because it was incomprehensible.

As much as possible, my goal was to keep our lives on a normal schedule. This probably reflected my own denial, shock, and stubbornness. Nonetheless, our family was constrained so much by this illness that I wanted to retake control. Anorexia is a syndrome of control—the control of a lying, deceitful terrorist. A brain's attempt to control *hard to feel* feelings! I didn't want to avoid public places because of Terrorist Joey. I didn't want to concede my time, my son's time, our family values and interests because this monster said so. This was my way of fighting back and trying to restore a functioning home.

My friend Loren texted me that she wanted to get together. She knew of Brother's illness, and she was also a therapist on the island who was providing me emotional support and encouragement. We decided to meet up for church Sunday morning, and then she followed us home to carpool for an afternoon at the beach. We wanted to maximize sun time so I chose to pack picnic lunches. Because of the packed schedule I kept, the traffic patterns, and the mobile life we led, the reality was that sometimes eating was on the run. Within our new normal, I knew this was a calculated risk, but we went ahead anyway. I made hotdogs on a bun with condiments, fruit, chips, and portable drinks to go. I drove, Loren shotgun, with both of my boys in the rear, and I handed back the food. As we started off, we immediately hit a detour...two ladies and a garage sale sign. It was fate. Loren and I looked at each other and laughed. I didn't have the heart to say, *You know what? Even this small change may upset Brother.*

I expected that our life was going forward and so would Brother's. I encouraged Loren to get started shopping, and I said I would join her after Brother finished his hotdog. He was never left unmonitored with food. That was rule number one! She got out and I turned around. Brother had tears spilling out of his eyes and a grip on his hotdog that rivaled an arm wrestling match. He was squeezing as tight as possible and shaking. It fell into pieces all over his lap and the backseat floor. Ketchup and mustard included. My determination matched his own and I declared that he would have to eat two hotdogs still—this had been his first. I wouldn't be deterred by mangled messes. So I handed him his second hotdog. He locked tearful eyes with my determined ones and started to squeeze again. I covered his hand with mine, and with firm intent, I told him he would be eating it regardless of where it landed and no matter how dirty it was.

I intercepted this hotdog from falling, centimeters from the seat, and handed it back to him. It was limp and in pieces, but edible and clean. I placed it in a Tupperware bowl and told him to eat. This demand was momentous and the context intense. He was fighting with himself in his head. I jokingly remind my kids often that I cannot read minds, but if I ever could, I swear this moment was it. It was like watching a mental play by play with Joey versus Brother; who would win this round? I could imagine Joey's sinuous rasp telling Brother that he would feel better if he didn't eat, and food was bad, and his mother was just trying to make him fat. Joey surely whispered to Brother that he was weak if he ate and that he deserved this misery. Brother's eyes shone with fear and distress, illuminating this internal battle.

The surf was his motivation, so my ultimatum was to turn around and return home. Again, my determined stance was not meant in meanness but in advocacy. If Brother could concede to me—his authority figure—then Joey was at least fighting a healthy brain and not a malnourished, self-defeating one. It wasn't a matter of willpower. Brother had incredible willpower and had proven that more than anyone I had ever known! It was, however, certainly a matter of control, distortion, and extortion. My battle line was drawn, and I was doing everything I could to bring Brother back to my side. He forced that hotdog down, bite by bite, and needless to say, I never joined Loren at the garage sale. I gave him a second hotdog, this one mine, and he choked it down as well. He ended up with every single bite he would have had without this episode, just as I had intended. We traveled on toward the beach, and both boys successfully completed their meals. Brother was allowed to surf for a short while as Loren and I decompressed.

Our culture is saturated with emphasis on body image, fitness, and health. Many people have asked me why this happened to my son. I have a complex answer involving many variables, not the least of which being that the world he has been raised in is obsessed with body image; we see evidence of it in nearly every commercial, movie, mall, magazine rack, and even doctor's office. Until I was tasked with sheltering an anorexic teen from the words *health* and *thin*, I had not truly realized the bombardment and impact of these subtle and not so subtle messages everywhere one turns.

One example is the emphasis in athletic circles about body types. Since a very young age, Brother has been interested in sports, and throughout his childhood, he has participated in organized teams for soccer, football, baseball, and basketball. His leisure time interests have consistently revolved around ESPN and sport video games. Those games allow a person to choose the body type of the athlete in the virtual world or input the real life measurements of the actual athlete to simulate plays that parallel real life capabilities. Stats and comparisons of body types are normalized and expected. These messages are subtle, yet to an intuitive kid, they send the message that being athletic and "good enough" correlates to body type. And to add to those indirect societal messages was a direct and troubling memory.

When Brother was age eleven or so, he had participated on a tackle football team for the first time. The season seemed to be going smoothly, and Brother was part of a very successful team. However, one day I recalled as he was getting on his uniform in preparation for a game, he had pointed to a sticker on his helmet and said, "That's a *fat sticker*, Mom." Taken aback, I responded, "What!?" He explained that his coach had given some of the kids *fat stickers* if they were not allowed to play certain positions because of their weight and that he had passed the cutoff for those positions by a pound or two. I was appalled at this labeling and countered to my son that by *no means* was he fat. I was rather ignorant about coaching methods, but regardless of the coach's rationale, I reassured Brother he was a very healthy, normal weight for his age and stature. Even though in some football positions the benefits of a larger frame are promoted, *fat* as a label has a negative connotation, and in this instance, it had a prohibitive consequence. Certainly, it could be argued that this unnecessary labeling experience in Brother's early preteen years was a contributing culprit to his later development of body image issues.

Now, as a parent with a child diagnosed with anorexia, living in a society that promoted health as thinness, I realized that even good messages can be internalized in destructive ways. I was sensitive and perceptive to the underlying messages about body types, even those that were prosocial in intent. Case in point, I took Brother to his medical appointment early in his emaciated state and I recall scanning the posters in the waiting room and realizing how pervasive the topic of food is, as the food pyramid stared back at me and images of children being *active* and eating *healthy* leaped out at me from the images depicted. Then my eyes caught the title of a brochure in one of those plastic cubbies and I reached for it: *How to feed your adolescent child* it read. Great, the very topic I need! And then, bam, several pages of how to eat in moderation, what not to eat, and what to avoid, all sending the message to help your child manage his/her weight and, ultimately, *not get fat.*

How do children filter all this? They have to receive in many ways, over many days, the hidden message that *Fat is bad.* For the public majority, these messages help curb impulses, encourage healthy eating choices, and explain how to live a balanced lifestyle. Yet for a perfectionistic minded minority, like my son, this message is interpreted as, *Well, if fat is bad, then I won't be fat and fail at dieting like all those people I see in the world around me.* He assimilated this value system before he had the mental awareness and maturity to determine whether it was his own value system. He was doing what he legitimately thought was right, in his best interest, and would bring him happiness because our society was cramming this value system down his throat.

Product marketing does this incessantly. *Here is what's wrong with you*, they say, *and here is what I can offer you to fix that...for this price.* My frustration increased as I had conversation after conversation with people over the next few months who, unaware of my son's struggle with food, made casual comments such as, "I ate a cookie, and now I have to run a mile," and "I really need to lose these last few pounds." I can bet a fat load of cash, pun intended, you have heard this topic come up in casual conversation at least once this week, probably daily. It is everywhere! To be fat is perceived as being a personal failure, and discrimination against full body shapes abounds in our culture. On every playground where young moms struggle to regain their pre-baby body, on every sports team, in every gym, in every school hallway, in every school lunchroom, in military chow halls, on every Facebook page, in every family tree, in most every New Year's resolution, and certainly in the hijacked mind of my precious boy. Don't get fat, or stay fat, or...*what*? Be unlovable. Unaccepted. *Isn't that part of the underlying fear?* I hate this societal message, and I bristled against it as I was bombarded with the realization of how pervasive it truly is. In my frustration, I wanted to scream at every person who used the word *fat* or talked about *working out* or *dieting*. These words were potentially deadly in our home.

Deep connection is the antidote to madness.

— Stefan Molyneux

CHAPTER 12

LOSING LOGIC

Another group meal drop off for Brother. Two hours of sanity for me. And a rare chance to connect individually with my youngest son.

We drove home to fix our own meal and complete homework and chores in general. The brief time Brother was at group was one of the only opportunities outside of their sleep time when I could catch up on home duties, grocery shopping, or other errands, and have some mental reprieve from the unpredictable mood shifts of the anorexic mind.

I looked in my rearview mirror, grateful not to have to explain myself in this simple movement, and I asked my youngest how he was doing with all of this madness. I will never forget his response. With voice trembling and tears threatening to spill over his cheeks, he said he was worried that he was going to "get this too" when he was older. He added, "I don't want to lose my logic like Brother did."

Perfectly said!

Got to love the honesty that comes out of a child's mouth! He voiced his reasonable fears given what he knew of the world at age nine, and I was given the opportunity to assuage them. I explained how this illness was not contagious and very rare, especially for boys, and how watching his brother go through this horrible experience would likely protect him from ever dealing with this in his own life. I explained to him that his brother didn't ask for this situation, didn't deserve it, but, like cancer, it had happened to him. However, this wasn't a normal part of growing up.

My son seemed relieved to hear this, and then he made a wise statement well beyond his years. "Mom, it's okay because he is going to help people someday because of this," my precious youngest stated with certainty. "Maybe he'll be a counselor like you and maybe not, but he will help other people who are going through this," he added.

A lump caught in my throat as my pride threatened to spill over. What youthful confidence that paralleled my own belief in the likely outcome after *this too had passed*. It was optimism I desperately clung to. I know my children. I know their personalities and their passions and how they relate to others. Brother is a conscientious, compassionate, empathetic soul who is driven, perfectionistic, mindful, and task-oriented. He sets goals and achieves them. Clearly. This was evident in his ability to set the goal to starve and deny his body the basic primal needs of food and drink, which he did with good intentions (to feel better), yet without understanding the destructive impact it would have on his body and mind. He accomplished it, though. Somehow, over the course of seven weeks, he had ignored hunger cues, stomach pangs, and fought through the urge to respond to his appetite, meal after meal, hour after hour, and minute after minute. Most of us couldn't accomplish this for one day. He proved capable of impulse control beyond most of our wildest imaginations! Anorexia is not a disorder of appetite; it is a disorder of body image. So he felt hunger, just as you and I feel hunger. He was clearly a focused person with the ability to accomplish anything he put his mind to. My goal, and his younger brother's prediction, was to find a way to circumvent this tragic trajectory and find meaning in this pain.

Logic was indeed lost. Brain power is thinking power. Our brains require fat to function. Brain matter is literally made of fat cells! Roughly two-thirds of our cerebral cortex is comprised of the macronutrient fat. Ever hear of the term "essential fatty acids"? The term "essential" is a clue for how important these nutrients, especially Omega-3, obtained purely through diet, are. Deficiencies here severely restrict brain functioning by slowing down and deteriorating neurons' ability to send and receive messages, which is vital for mental health. On a cellular level, the cause and effect of restrictive eating includes sluggish thinking, memory problems, lethargy, moodiness, anxiety, irritability, and a depressed demeanor. (8)

Sluggish thinking became a life-altering handicap for Brother, and it was very evident to me in the early stages of his illness. I recall with great clarity his inability to solve a simple math problem during the first few months he was back at home. To top it off, he was literally unable to write clearly and legibly either. His handwriting appeared to be that of a first grader. As a result of his status with the school district he was placed on a pass/fail expectation with the school. Even this proved too high a mountain to scale as he averaged scores around 5 percent in many of his core classes.

Let me paint you a contextual picture. This was a child who, since second grade, had been chosen by recommendation of his teachers and test scores to be in the talented and gifted classes. He had never experienced academic failure. He had never struggled with comprehension or completion of tasks in this way. He was reading before kindergarten, became fluent in the German language by the age of seven, and received a letter of appreciation from the school district superintendent in fifth grade for his extremely high test scores in math, with a remark that the head honcho would like to "clone" him. This was an exceptionally gifted mind, hijacked and ransacked.

I am not an M.D., but I am an eyewitness. A witness to the reality that brain power requires nutrition—enough nutrition to set the sparks in motion long enough to saturate the cells and replenish the body with electrical charges that equate to being able to compute 50 x 3. If this nutrient supply is cut off too long, the result is disastrous. Most parents have been taught to *pick your battles*. That is essentially how I handled this particular symptom. Academics became a non-issue and merely a measuring stick of what had happened to this child under the layer of tissue we call skin—in the hidden crevices of a skeletal system that became more skeletal than system. My focus in a matter of days had shifted from enrolling him in school to enrolling him in a psychiatric eating disorder unit. My worry then shifted from "Will he miss school?" to "Will he pass eighth grade?" and landed somewhere in *who cares land*, where as long as he breathed and produced sweat and lifted a fork to his mouth, I was tickled pink! Everything trivial dissipates in this world with anorexia. What does matter when your child is ravaged by a terrorist from the inside out? What does a grade of "A" mean when your son is unable to sit on a couch because the imprint of his body convulses him in emotional pain?

This too was a troubling symptom. I mentioned obsessive compulsive movements and, along with the pacing, excessive standing, refusing to lean back into a chair, zigzag walking, grabbing his body around the legs and arms, checking their size, and sprinting, he also began to have a strange posture when approaching the dining room chair to sit. He would gingerly sit without applying pressure to the surface, quickly rise, then gingerly initiate sitting again. Then before he had landed, he would quickly rise and repeat this pattern for the count of what seemed to be five attempts before he would eventually sit. And when he finally sat, he would sit on the front edge of the seat and only on the side corner of the area. He appeared to be trying not to *feel* his body weight on the hard or soft surface, and he intended to use as little of the chair as humanly possible to support his frame.

I believe Brother wrongly interpreted evidence of his body on a chair in two ways: 1) taking up space (*any space*) was evidence of perceived fatness, and 2) the imprint or displacement of fabric meant he was fat. He would cry when this happened. He would stand or lay on the floor most of the time because that didn't move under his nominal weight. A couple of other household items betrayed his mind in this way. I had bought a kitchen sink mat that had memory foam in the interior. When I asked whether he liked it since it was new to the home, he said, "No" because he could see his foot imprint, and this bothered him, so he avoided this rug. He would stand next to it or behind it, not on it. The other item was a lounge chair that had wooden peg legs and was positioned on a linoleum floor. Sometimes when sitting in this chair or even accidently bumping against it without much force at all, it would move and shift on the ground. This bothered him immensely and would create one of his emotional episodes.

Let me expand on that further. These episodes varied in intensity and specifics during the course of his illness, but they always involved emotional release, catastrophic thinking, exaggeration, and perception errors. He would cry and repeat negative self-statements, sometimes with an incessant repetition, and fall into a state of inconsolable grief. Often, he would barrage me with questions about his body and demand I confirm his thoughts. I had been instructed by his treatment team to ignore these statements and respond with something like: "You know we are not going to talk about your body like you're a piece of fish," or "We don't talk about superficial things in this house," or "You are a vessel of God and your importance is internal." Then I would just walk away if necessary, ignoring the attempts to engage in this cyclical downward spiral.

Although these responses were important, they were hard to implement when my child was pleading with me incessantly to respond to his statement that, "I am fatter than I was before" *(as he compared himself to the person that got on that flight to New Mexico pre-summer)* or "fatter than I used to be" *(as he seemed determined to stay in a non-growing state)* and demanded confirmation that he was "not skinny."

I wanted to reassure him when he was being deceived. I wanted to shout, "You *are* skinny!" Dangerously skinny. I wanted desperately to delve into explaining body development, yet I had to stop myself and ignore these pleas for the time being. The belief here was that to offer platitudes would relieve the anxiety of the feeling fat for a brief moment, but it would reinforce this fixation on body evaluation. In summary, if you feed Terrorist Joey, he grows in power. If you deny him this mental food, he grows weaker. Terrorist Joey wanted confirmation that he was skinny. He wanted to be able to rub into Brother's psyche, "See, you feel better when you are skinny and people say so." This was the anxiety cycle. I longed to relieve his anxiety, but I knew to do so would only reinforce his mental state of defining his self-worth solely by his body measurements.

> ***TIP #12:*** *Do NOT respond to the endless pleas for reassurance about body image concerns. Ignore them. Do not reinforce the need to be evaluated by external measures that have no connection to the child's inherent value and worth. Respond with, "I know this is hard and I love you," or "This family does not engage in body talk." Walk away if necessary and use avoidance rather than conceding to the barrage.*

Anything that's human is mentionable,
and anything that is mentionable can be more
manageable. When we can talk about our feelings,
they become less overwhelming, less upsetting,
and less scary. The people we trust with that important
talk can help us know that we are not alone.

— Fred Rogers

CHAPTER 13

THE TIDE SHIFTS

"That's okay, Mom, I'll just wear my T-shirt." A statement that stopped me in my tracks as I prepared the kids for bed and gathered up their clothing piles for the next morning.

It was Tuesday evening, October 1, and since I had laid eyes on Brother after the terrorist invasion, on July 27, he had refused to take off his cover to the world—his sweatshirt. It was a constant companion, despite the hot, clammy days of Hawaii in the fall. He was never seen without one, so this statement seemed momentous. His wardrobe had adjusted to his condition, and the clothes I had bought him in anticipation of a new school year still lay folded or hung unused. The only thing he had been able to wear were gym shorts and his school uniform shirt with a sweatshirt to hide under. Nothing with a waistline, or he would have flipped out, and feeling form fitted fabric on his skin could trigger an avalanche of *feel fat fears*.

"What was that?" my heart quickened as I questioned, hoping I had heard correctly. "It's okay, Mom, if you don't want to find me a sweatshirt, *I guess*," he said, trying to sound nonchalant.

"All right then," I happily responded and kissed him good night. Outside the door, under the protective cloak of privacy, I cried. A flood of unstoppable tears of relief.

Brother's eventual willingness to shed his outer wardrobe layer was indicative of his internal temperature regulator coming out of sleep mode. This was evidence he was finally uncomfortable in the heat, even though he was unwilling verbally to acknowledge that fact. Fans are required household appliances when you live in Hawaii and our home was no exception. When I finally saw Brother starting to sweat, I realized that our small clan had need of another fan because, like it or not, I was going to place one in the vicinity of Brother while he slept, despite his adamant stance that he "didn't want one." His thinking was that admitting he gets hot at night was paramount to admitting he was overweight because he equated sweating with obesity. His thinking error was *only fat people sweat,* and he did not want to identify with *fat*, so his discomfort as he slept was more acceptable than admitting this perceived body image failure. Hence began a very memorable shopping trip to a local hardware store.

Because of our new normal, I always seemed to be rushing around in a frenzy and this day was no exception. Ambitiously, I planned to buy the fan and then go on a secret underwear buying mission, convinced if I got Brother undergarments one size larger, he might ease back into his skin with a shade less anxiety and angst. So I gathered up my purchase items from the first stop and shepherded my two less than pleased children to the checkout register. My boys are like most others their age; they detest errands, and shopping is a double negative.

After paying for my items, I reverted back to my old mom mode (the self before anorexia invaded) and asked my normally compliant oldest to hold the fan for me while I managed my purse and other small bagged purchases. He begrudgingly allowed me to place the box, which was probably all of three pounds, in his arms, and we began walking to the car. As I walked, I looked back, checking on his progress. I was stunned to see the box slowly slipping out of his hands as he leaned over as if he were carrying lead weights strapped to his midsection—with his exaggerated posture sending the wordless message that this task was beyond his ability.

Surprised, I quickly intercepted the falling fan box and held it up with a puzzled expression. Brother complained, "I can't!" with an edge of irritation and began crying. He was visibly distressed, and I realized, there in the parking lot, the extent to which Terrorist Joey had convinced him that *strength* was *fat*, and therefore, *strength was bad*. To admit he was able to carry a three pound box for his mother was on par with accepting fatness in his delusional state of mind.

As he shook and cried I continued walking to the car and placed the box in the trunk. Then I looked directly at him and stated that this was an expected task for someone of his age. It was not a sign of being fat or overweight, it was a sign of being alive and healthy enough to hold an object. He disagreed and shook his head dismissively and accusatorily stated, "You think I'm fat. You think I can carry that!"

It was such a surreal moment because it would have been absurdly comical if we didn't live with Terrorist Joey. With determination, I chose to shake it off and march our small troop into the next store. I knew I couldn't leave Brother alone in the car with mirrors, but taking him into the department store with mirrors was equally daunting. The upside was I'd be there to watch him. So we went to a retail store with the intent to covertly sneak underwear to the counter. He made it only a few aisles in before he grabbed his stomach and whimpered that he was fat. He had caught a glimpse of himself in the aisle mirrors, which triggered his anorexic thoughts. In exasperation, I corralled him to a non-reflective part of the store and instructed him to sit and wait while I ran to the aforementioned department. With the underwear purchase hidden in the cart and now questioning the wisdom of my choice, we exited as quickly as humanly possible. This one small task was emotionally draining and telling of how severe his life dysfunction had become under the reign of Joey's terror.

From July to early October, I could not touch my son—couldn't get anywhere near him, or he would withdraw and retract like a sea anemone. He wouldn't sit down unless forced, couldn't stop anxious pacing, wouldn't move without being told to, had to be prompted to sit, wouldn't lean back in his chair when he did sit, and wouldn't recline in his bed when reading or otherwise until the final moment before succumbing to sleep. He was tired all the time, could not think, showed serious cognitive deficits and problem solving constraints, and decision making proved nearly impossible. He was constipated and complained of stomach pain at every meal and between meals. He complained so many times that I made calls to his pediatrician to make sure he wasn't having some intestinal complications. His mantra was *"I can tell!" "I can tell I am bigger than I was before!"* This was repeated daily at the frequency of...well, a repeat button on a CD that never seems to end.

He would touch his legs and his arms, holding them up and looking them over or encircling his fingers around them to estimate size. I would see him hike up his shorts to assess his thighs on a regular basis. He could only stand loose clothing and would only wear sandals, not shoes, because the latter felt restrictive—aka fat—on his feet. He was a prisoner in his body and head. Food and nourishment were the keys to his release. During this time, he had to be told when to wipe his face and when not to wipe his face. He did not laugh, nor smile, nor show any social interest. He directly stated he didn't want to make friends, was listless, lethargic, and could not be left alone at all. Starving equaled depressed. Think back to any movie you have seen that depicted concentration camp victims. How did they act? How did they move? How did they seem?

This was my son's life in essence...what he was diminished to.

That year, fall break at school was from October 7 to 11. It provided a naturally occurring opportunity for trial and error with Brother's monitoring regimen. Per his nutritionist, it was time to see whether he was able to manage eating lunch on his own. There were concerns he would skip lunch altogether. Apprehensions he would take minimal portions or purge if he did eat. Nonetheless, he needed to be allowed incremental control back into his eating world. The treatment team and I agreed on a plan to give eating with peers in the lunchroom a try after this break.

As planned, Brother was able to eat with his peers in the lunchroom when he returned to school after fall break. I still sent packed lunches so I would at least know what food he went into the lunchroom with, and a packed lunch was less overwhelming for him than to have to pick an entree and sides and be entrusted with all those tasks. The school counselor promised to watch out for him and relay observations, but I was instructed by his nutritionist not to ask him directly how he ate—the premise being if he restricted or did not consume his food, he would feel guilt and be tempted to lie to cover that emotion, thereby, setting off a vicious shame cycle.

It was terribly hard to comply with this advice, but I did and trusted that the truth would be told through the scale. The first two reports were saddening but hopeful. Brother was sitting alone and not interacting with others, but at least he had food on his tray and was using his meal card, as the balance was proving. Things seemed to go well for the first week or two, but then I got a call from Angel Kirsten with a report that Brother had been seen sitting with a family friend and not eating at all. Also during lunch club, which Angel Kirsten and her husband organized and led every Wednesday at the school, he had been seen with food in his lunchbox one minute, but all of it had disappeared by the next. Presumed dumping. Plus he had returned home with nothing to show in his lunchbox except the freezer ice packets. Baggies and all were gone, which was unusual.

That triggered a confrontational talk and I fessed up to my insider knowledge and, despite his denial of all of the above, I explained that regardless of whether dumping had happened or not, he was going back to counselor-monitored lunches. For now. This was not regression. It was prevention. He needed more hand-holding, so to speak, and I did not believe I should ask his permission for that. It just had to happen. He went back to the monitored system, yet I explained it would only remain for a couple of weeks before he was given an opportunity again. I needed him to know it was a trust system and that trust could be earned. Still, he was insistent that he wanted more control over his food. And he complained adamantly that he was *never* going to be trusted again, *never* going to leave group, *never* going to be able to eat alone, and *never* __________ (fill in the blank). You name it. He was dejected and pessimistic. Reassurance was given, and yet structure, consistency, and firmness, with compassion, were the tools most used.

Guidance at this time from his dietician was immensely helpful. She advised me to begin giving him choices for which foods to have for meals, as long as those options were controlled and all met the prescriptive meal plan criteria. He could then decide on whole milk or juice, bread or rice, chicken or beef, cheese or ranch sauce—all within the backdrop of making sure all options totaled his required caloric intake. He responded well to this and, as long as the menu changed frequently, he wasn't allowed to confine himself to certain foods over others.

That was still his tendency. He would avoid any and all condiments with intense kickback if he was expected to consume them. He said things like, "I have never liked that" regarding foods that he had surely eaten in times past with enjoyment. Butter, specifically. Tearful tantrums ensued when he discovered butter on his bread. Or salt sprinkled on his peas. He wanted fish and vegetables and fruit only. Plain. No ketchup, mustard, ranch, tartar sauce, or vinaigrette. He requested salad when he had never willingly eaten salad before. And holy smokes, an avalanche of tears if I put salad dressing on the dry leaf bed!

He avoided cheese at all costs and wanted plain yogurt, nixing the granola. So the delicate balance became offering a smorgasbord of ever-changing options, always intentionally involving something his brain wanted to avoid. Again, it wasn't about the food itself. It was the fear behind it.

Soda was the forbidden fruit and the most taboo of taboos. It was also the first identifiable restrictive behavior, in hindsight, even before anorexia entered the scene. In the beginning, it seemed to be a smart choice. One that was respected and supported. He had made the decision for New Year's of 2012 to give up soda. He just didn't believe it was good for him, and he didn't need it. Nowhere in that decision did he or I see the glaring headlights of anorexia moving slowly down the road in our direction. It was just that. Giving up soda. He didn't starve himself. He didn't deny hunger pangs. It was an isolated decision, yet perhaps an interesting precursor. Certainly, this child had incredible impulse control and had proven so even in his youth in that very innocent decision. The day came, therefore, when soda was a weapon in my arsenal against Joey. Orange crush at L and L Hawaiian Barbeque drive-in. This was the hardest thing for me to do. I felt like I was betraying Brother, but I had to make him drink it. He fought it. The tears tried to win. The pleas tried to change my mind. Yet even in this mini-battle, I felt it was me against Joey, and the prize was my son's life. Soda didn't matter anymore. New Year's resolutions didn't matter anymore. The only thing that did was health. And health came in the form of a sugary, caffeinated drink with chemicals I can't even spell.

> ***TIP #13:*** *Do not aid and abet the food "taboo" list. Make sure the anorexic's meal plan includes the very foods they wish to avoid. It's the mental resistance you are targeting.*

If you believe anorexics choose not to eat, you talk and rage and sometimes give up. If you believe they can't eat, you lovingly make the decision for them until they can.

— Laura Collins, *Eating with Your Anorexic*

CHAPTER 14

WHAT IS MAUDSLEY?

Brother's treatment was implemented primarily with the principles of the Maudsley treatment approach, developed in the Maudsley Hospital in London. These concepts were the first I encountered in my online search, and their targeted approach fit my clinical understanding and seemed to provide some answers to what I *could* and *needed* to do. They were reinforced by the majority of specialists from whom I sought advice. According to Dr. Angela Celio Doyle with the University of Chicago's Eating Disorder Program:

> The treatment involves compassionate, yet persistent and firm expectations that your adolescent eat an amount of food that can reverse the state of starvation his or her body is in and help them gain weight. Due to the nature of anorexia nervosa, which causes an adolescent to truly fear the effects of food and weight gain, anorexic adolescents will

resist eating—especially the amounts and kinds of foods that are necessary for weight gain. In these situations, professional treatment assists parents in determining how to make the three meals and three snacks per day happen in a compassionate and successful way. Some families encounter a moderate amount of resistance from their adolescent during meals and some encounter a lot—hearing stories from other families about their experiences can be helpful in depicting the variations in how this "looks" for any particular family. Working with a professional trained in the Maudsley approach will help to determine the best way to address the resistance to eating.

Maudsley is not punitive in any way and involves quite a bit of emotional support. Some parents may fear that they are being insensitive to their adolescent if they "push" their child to eat a plate of Fettuccine Alfredo when the adolescent is refusing, crying, or otherwise resisting. However, if you consider a child or adolescent with a chronic illness, such as cancer, who pleads with their parent to avoid another bout of chemotherapy because it makes them feel sick, a parent would compassionately, yet firmly, determine that the chemotherapy is needed, despite how it makes them feel. In this way, some parents of adolescents with anorexia find it helpful to view food as "medicine" for their child's illness that is required to, quite literally, save their life. It is also important to remember that the resistance to

> eating stems from the anorexia, not the healthy, wonderful child who was overtaken by this illness. Understanding that the anorexia is separate from your adolescent may help in remembering that you are helping your child while eliminating the anorexia nervosa through increasing calorie consumption. (9)

Doctors Daniel Le Grange, Ph.D., and James Lock, M.D., Ph.D., are top experts in researching and treating this medical condition, and they describe the Maudsley intervention in the following manner:

> The Maudsley approach can mostly be construed as an intensive outpatient treatment where parents play an active and positive role in order to: Help restore their child's weight to normal levels expected given their adolescent's age and height; hand the control over eating back to the adolescent, and; encourage normal adolescent development through an in-depth discussion of these crucial developmental issues as they pertain to their child. (10)

I took these renowned doctors' guidance to heart, and the books and scholarly articles penned by them were a lifeline I held on to and a GPS for our everyday living. This evidence-based treatment method has been demonstrated in clinical studies to help approximately two-thirds of participating teens diagnosed with anorexia nervosa to beat this illness by the end of a twelve-month period. And the statistics suggest those gains last, since the majority of those triumphant teens remain weight-restored at follow-up five years post-treatment. Early intervention is extremely important as the time in illness seems correlated to treatment prognosis. The Maudsley method has a proven track record with patients who have been sick a comparatively short length of time, ideally a span of no more than three years from diagnosis until intervention. (11)

> ***TIP #14:*** *Consider the Maudsley Approach: Family Based Treatment as an empirically validated intervention for helping your child beat his or her eating disorder. The sooner treatment is sought, the better.*

Strength, a river cuts through a rock not
because of its power but its persistence.

– Jim Watkins

CHAPTER 15

IN THE ZONE

My faith is my rock. Church attendance during this time was critical to my spiritual sanity. One Sunday morning late in October, as we were driving home from this sanctuary, Brother asked, *"Can I have some water, Mom?"* Mind you, had my body been hooked up to an EKG machine, it surely would have showed my heart skipped a beat.

To put this request in context, it had been more than two months since his hospitalization, four months since I have normal memories of eating patterns with this child, and he had not once initiated *any* semblance of food or liquid intake. He only ate because hospital staff or I required him to. He only drank water when a caregiver handed it to him. Even these instances filled him with angst and resulted in complaining.

As I handed him the water bottle, I realized that he was responding to real, strong thirst after having played a game of soccer with some church buddies. A moment or two later, I would have handed him the bottle myself with the instruction that he drink, but he had beaten me to it!

It amazes me how I continued to keep my hands on the wheel and maneuver that block of machinery when my mind and heart were racing. This was HUGE. This was a legitimate, self-initiated request for body nourishment—for that life-giving source called water. When we arrived home, my glee continued as he went to the faucet and filled a second glass of water! Joy, pure joy! Had I never traveled this road, I would never have known the ecstasy of watching one's child drink when thirsty and understanding truly what that meant internally. Terrorist Joey score eight million and Brother score one at that moment. Healing was happening! Upon arriving home, I immediately texted the Angels in our life, unable to contain my happiness over this monumental step. Good news was meant to be shared. They rejoiced with me.

Within weeks of Brother's water triumph, I heard the blessed phrase: *"I like Maui Mike's; we haven't eaten there in a while."* This was the first food statement I had heard from my son. The month of October held some extreme highs and extreme lows in his fight for sanity. I would have moved mountains to get him to Maui Mikes. Instead, I just had to move my schedule, my body, and the car into gear. Simple!

We were on the way that very weekend. It was like feasting in heaven. Maui Mike's is a rotisserie chicken eatery in the town of Wahiawa on Oahu, despite its name. Its fire-roasted chicken satisfies tourists and locals alike, and it had quickly become our family's tradition en route to the north shore when we would venture out that way. It was an hour drive one way, but oh, so worth it! I ordered the *small feast* with Brother's favorite *lava hot* sauce and my favorite teriyaki dip and settled in to a messy, finger-licking delight. This meal was extra great not because of the chicken itself, but the meaning behind it. Finally, it was acceptable in Brother's head to say out loud that he wanted food. And specific food even. He had a positive attitude and ate willingly, yet the tendency was still there to avoid eating all the chicken and not so many pieces. So I gently encouraged him, chicken leg by chicken thigh, until the only thing left to do was lick our fingers. Oh, so *ono* (Hawaiian for *good*).

Several things can be credited for the progress we were seeing. One was his quick weight gain. He was blind-weighed (meaning he could not see the scale) every week in his nutritionist's office, and each week he made his weight gain goal for that period.

We never had a stagnant week because Terrorist Joey never had a chance to restrict food secretly. Monitoring of Brother's eating was so thorough and complete that weight gain was inevitable. From start to finish during his treatment, his body needed to pack on thirty-six pounds to be *in the zone* (a healthy target range for his height, gender, and age, based on his own early childhood growth charts).

Brother had lost one third of his body composition and had to regain that one third back. Through grit, determination, and unwavering resolve, this goal was accomplished in approximately ten weeks. That's an average of four pounds a week. Break it down meal by meal and it was nothing short of a miracle. Each calorie and pound represented climbing an emotional and physical mountain and making it to the top. Each number on the scale represented an adult in Brother's life sitting down with him and watching, talking, caring, supporting, and keeping him accountable. Each hash mark on the chart indicated one huge stroke against Terrorist Joey and one giant leap of progress for Brother and mental health. Each one of those for me was a very personal and serious "Take that Joey; get out of Brother's life for good" message.

Remember, the three-step process to recovery with this illness that our treatment team had preached: weight restoration, addressing body image and psychological issues, and then family dynamics. Many people never make it to phase two, and for those who do, the journey is often long and spread out across too great a timespan. I recall the moment I heard Brother's nutritionist say he was "in the zone." It was like being told Brother had won the lottery—of life. But what did that mean? It meant he weighed *enough*. Enough not to shiver as he lay in the hot climate of Hawaii in fall. Enough to sweat again. Enough to sit down without feeling pain (if only his mind would let him). Enough not to appear to the general public as though he was a concentration camp survivor.

Yet there were two phases to go. The *exterior* was repaired, but the *interior* was in shambles. What Brother had not regained was the ability to smile, to think, to choose life—and food. The ability to concentrate, to manage his moods, to see himself truly as he was. The awareness that he looked good, and the ability to accept it.

Psychiatric medication was a topic visited occasionally. This was first introduced as an option in the hospital, and our parental stance on it was *avoid if possible but use if necessary*. The psychiatrist there was a drug minimalist, much to my liking, and therefore, we did not cross this bridge until later in the treatment process. The nutritionist and psychiatrist we were working with on the island explained to me that due to Brother's increasing levels of anxiety and compulsive behaviors, he was a good candidate for medication intervention. They explained that, nearly without exception, all of their clients were managed medically using psychotropic drugs and with great success in mitigating the intensity of the feel fat thoughts, and it *took the edge off* their struggle.

Well, we needed *something* to take the edge off, and I was desperate to do anything to help ease his mental anguish, so we began a course of Lexapro. He started on five milligrams, which was increased to ten milligrams after three days, and then, after two weeks of believed drug toleration, the dose was increased to fifteen milligrams.

The first two weeks of drug intervention seemed to have a small but noticeable effect on his anxiety levels. If they were at a ten, they dropped to an eight or so on the scale. Small but helpful! However, a couple of days after increasing the dose five more milligrams, I received a concerning call from Brother's caregiver. My friend, Angel Kirsten, calmly shared that after school she had been helping Brother with his homework and sitting with him at their family dining room table when a random and unexpected conversation took place. Apparently, my child stopped mid-task, looked her directly in the eyes, and calmly stated: *"Mass shooting. I think you want to die. I should kill you."* Stunned but composed, she responded, *"Well, actually, I don't want to die, and I am sure I want to live,"* at which point he became quiet, then dropped his glance, and went back to his task.

How does a parent process a call like that? I asked her what his demeanor was like. She described it as strange and mentally absent, as if it were his voice talking, but he wasn't aware of it. A seemingly out-of-mind experience. I didn't know what to do. We discussed how to handle this. Then I thanked her for bringing it to my attention and told her to please let me know whether anything *remotely* close to this happened again. My heart hoped it wouldn't and that it was some fluke—but reality bites hard. The very next day, he was riding in the car with me when he began talking about suicide and dying, passively commenting, "Well, I might as well die."

I am a trained mental health counselor, so I deal with the topic of suicide frequently with clients and take such comments seriously, and I told my son so. He denied any intent to follow through with such thoughts and tried to change the topic. I countered with my plan to get help if he were struggling with these thoughts, and I implored him to be honest with me. I also informed him that I was very concerned that he was saying or thinking such things and that I would be asking his caregivers to report to me any such occurrences. I already knew about his comments from the day prior, but I had not informed him of my knowledge. Angel Kirsten and I wanted to handle it delicately to foster his trust and rapport with her, rather than encourage the secrecy that suicidal thoughts usually wish to have.

As part of my crisis management plan, I contacted Angel Ingrid and received guidance and referral to a children's hospital that dealt with safety issues in case we needed to act immediately. I informed Brother's psychiatrist about his terrifying comments, but after speaking with Brother briefly, she seemed relatively unconcerned and recommended he continue on the medication. I proceeded according to her recommendation; however, two days later, I got hit with a déjà vu bomb. When picking up Brother after school, Angel Kirsten pulled me aside and said that it had happened again. This time was less direct, but Brother's comments involved dying and killing people. Emotionally devastated, I spent the rest of the evening pondering how to handle it.

I called Brother's dad and informed him of this recent development. We were both surprised since such thoughts had never occurred before to our knowledge. I recalled that even when reading Brother's inpatient paperwork and journaling, zero evidence existed of him wanting to hurt himself or anyone else even in his worst physical state.

Where is the manual that explains how parents start a conversation, casually, with their child about his threats to kill people? Who had anxiety now!

When Brother went to bed that evening, I followed, sat down at the edge of his bed, and explained what I had been told. His facial expression was telling. His eyebrows slanted in confusion, his neck cocked, his eyes teared up with sadness, and with a tremor in his voice, he asked, "Who heard that, Mom?" with a concerned tone full of worry. I explained that the only person who had heard him make that statement was Angel Kirsten. Relieved, he asked, "Were the kids around?" (Angel Kirsten has five children ranging in age from four to fourteen.)

Brother seemed completely unaware that he had said what he said!

"Um, no, they were not," I reassured him (as I had been assured earlier). With facial expression full of confusion, shame, and shock, he expressed genuine relief. Brother clearly did not want to hurt anyone! I had a serious conversation with him about my concerns that these kinds of statements were made. When I inquired directly whether he remembered saying them, he adamantly denied having any knowledge of the conversation taking place and, based on his body language and emotional reaction, I was convinced he was being truthful. We then had a very cautionary talk about the need to censor his words because, said in the wrong place, such as school, these words would have disastrous consequences for him and would be taken seriously by people who may not compassionately understand his condition. He nodded and appeared afraid, as if this situation was happening to him without his permission.

I followed up with Angel Ingrid regarding this recent episode and, based on her clinical knowledge and expertise, she adamantly and firmly recommended he be taken off the medication. As a therapist herself, she was knowledgeable about these types of reactions to medication, which can occur in anyone, but especially children.
She immediately consulted with another impartial psychiatrist, who confirmed the recommendation to pull him off his medication. Despite Brother's psychiatrist's assurance, I then made the parental choice to take him off Lexapro. I never gave him another dose after that day.

His anxiety did increase to the ten range again, so I knew we were going to have to battle that without chemical help. Help like that wasn't really help after all!

I am convinced this side effect for my son may not be the case for others. Psychiatric medication is a necessary thing for some people at the right dose with the right prescription. But this equation wasn't right for my son at that time, and therefore, I became leery to try another variant of the same. Without the enthusiastic support of Brother's psychiatrist and nutritionist, I, the parent, chose to do what I believed to be in the best interest of my son... which was implementing the Maudsley Approach Family Based Treatment...without the aid of medication. This approach may not be right for everyone in such circumstances—there is no cookie cutter healing equation—but I believe mothers have a sixth sense, and it is wise to follow your intuition. We never had to revisit this issue, and Brother eventually completed his treatment un-drugged. This seemed purely medication-induced and never reappeared after he was pulled off of them. No other self-harm or other harm comments were made. Thank you, Jesus.

TIP #15: *Discuss the pros and cons of psychotropic medication with your child's psychiatrist. Research the drug yourself and ask lots of questions. Pay attention to how your child is responding to the drug intervention if you go this route, and do not ignore your parental instinct.*

Tears are words the heart can't express.

— Gerard Way

CHAPTER 16

SOMETHING NOT QUITE HUMAN

Despite the physical progress, something unseen shifted again. Brother began regularly having animalistic moaning/screaming/wailing episodes numerous times a day. During the hours he was with me and not in school, they happened on average ten times daily, and they lasted for what seemed forever unless I was able to intervene. The sounds were guttural and raw, and I desperately recorded some of them on my phone in part to share with Angel Ingrid to get help, and in part, to have proof it happened because it seemed unworldly and surreal. I wish there was an audio clip inserted in this writing—that would be the only way to convey the intensity of those moments and the sounds I heard.

At one point, I called Angel Ingrid while the sounds were happening so she could bear witness and give guidance. She asked whether I felt safe, and for the first time, I could not answer, "Yes." I was terrified—for Brother, for my youngest, for myself. When she mentioned a psychotic break, this nearly made me have my own! No one wants this situation for his or her child. I wanted to crawl into a state of denial and plug my ears. One of the only things that seemed to moderate Brother's experience at all was to pull him in and hug him. A simple hug. He would lean in and place his head on my shoulder like he did many moons ago, and this seemed to provide some type of regressed comfort. His tiny frame would sink into mine, and he would seem to release his burden a little.

This stage made me feel my child was caught in a spiritual and emotional battle for his very life and sanity. There seemed to be an influential stranglehold on his life that was not his own. Because I believe people are spiritual, physical, mental, and emotional beings, I explored how to treat this behavior on all levels. I was already working the physical angle with the nutritionist and medical team, the emotional and mental angle with the psychiatrist, and the spiritual with my knees and my God. I was praying for Brother, but I needed backup. This behavior was otherworldly and required advanced weapons. I emailed my pastor and asked for his help.

He suggested we pray over Brother with the church elders between services the upcoming Sunday morning, which we did. We met and gathered at the front of the church behind the cover of the sound equipment and projection screen. Four brave men of God stood with us in a circle, placed their arms on our shoulders, and beseeched the throne of Jehovah Rapha, the God who heals.

My senses were on high alert, and through tears and fears, I felt and saw my son shrink under the church elders' touch—shrink and retract and try to avoid the encounter. Whether the sensation of touch was still painful and unbearable for him, I do not know. Whether it was a territorial reflex of the Evil One, I do not know. What I know is that he did try to avoid their touch; it was hard for Brother, but I am forever grateful for the elders' intercessory prayers and spiritual protection.

This stranglehold was thought-based and it was powerful, and it came out in physical form. Friday evening, October 25, Brother wanted to go to a youth event for church; since he would be under the watchful care of the youth leaders—who thankfully were also the family who cared for him in their home before and after school—I allowed it.

In retrospect, Brother wasn't ready for this social experience. In the two hours we were apart, he had an emotional breakdown and climbed a tree in front of at least one member of the group; while in the tree, he wailed, screamed, and howled like an animal in pain.

He was in pain! He couldn't keep it in for even two short hours. He was trying to communicate this pain, but as his weight increased, the pain had nowhere to go but to fester inside or come out in raw form.

This behavior frightened the girl who witnessed it, and it caused some serious issues within the home where Brother was being cared for.

In another episode, in an attempt to manage his rage, Brother walked outside the home of the family who cared for him and crawled under a windowsill to wail and moan and rocked his body back and forth in clear sorrow. Unknown to him, two children inside were hearing and reacting to his distress with some of their own. It scared them.

Brother's ability to manage himself was null. His awareness of his body position seemed to have disappeared also. He would bump into things, flail his arms and body in haphazard ways when wailing, and seem oblivious to people's presence around him. He regressed into some earlier childhood behaviors, such as *munching*—a sound he had made as a toddler when he'd had a blankie he would munch on.

He accompanied Angel Kirsten to a preschool event one day when school was not in session. As Angel Kirsten led the preschoolers in song and activity, she described to me afterward that in this setting it hit her—Brother was one of them. He acted like a three-year-old, ate like one, and had the emotional self-control of one. This wasn't a demeaning description said in insult...it was a realization of what this teenage boy was experiencing despite his chronological age and physical form. He had emotionally regressed to this level, and it was hard to witness it without deep sadness. Tears spilled from her caring eyes as she relayed this aha moment.

She could leave her four year old out of her sight longer than she could my adolescent son! If she became distracted for a moment by any one of the other six or more children who were always in the home, it was dangerous because he was unpredictable and capable of harm in his episodes of emotional pain. Obliviously, he would bump into things and people and dart out in the street and in front of pedestrians.

The darting was very strange. His movements seemed pressured, and he wouldn't walk normally anywhere; rather he would sprint. He would get out of the car and sprint to the door. He would get up from the table and spring to the next room. He would run around and between people like they were road cones. This behavior usually resulted in a tearful ending when he would say something like, "See, I'm slow!" and "I can't run!" or "I'm the slowest person there!" if there was even a miniscule hesitation in his movements. He was unreasonable in his self-assessment and constantly comparing himself to others. He didn't realize and couldn't accept that he had experienced a near-death event in his life and was recuperating physically and nowhere near his peak physical shape. However, he expected to be and demanded it of himself. It was a losing predicament that perpetuated the cycle of negativity within him.

The very next day, Saturday, October 26, Brother was invited to a previous baseball teammate's birthday party. Prior to his visit that summer to his father, he had been playing on the Hickam Air Force Base's baseball team and had wanted to participate in the tournament and end of season party. He had wrapped up the best season of his life yet and had become one of the team's top pitchers after just trying this position for the first time. He had been a star. The whole team had loved him. Now he hadn't seen this teammate since before the summer and yet, grasping at attempts for normalcy and to encourage his social interests again, I decided he would go to the birthday party.

His teammate's family was gracious and accommodating...but they didn't know our family's secret. They had last seen Brother in peak physical health. They didn't know the boy I dropped off that day had nearly died a slow death by starvation since they had last seen him. They didn't know why he stood all the time or hardly knew how to talk to his friend anymore. They certainly didn't know that we were in the midst of an epic battle that seemed to have no end. What they did know was that he didn't want birthday cake!

You see, I had fed him before dropping him off, so he wouldn't have an excuse not to eat by pretending he had eaten at the party. This was my rule of thumb. He was never allowed in the care of others unless they knew about his illness and could hold him accountable, or if they didn't know, I would alter his schedule so he would be with me during all feeding times.

That day he ate in the car on the way there and was mad at me for it. I am sure Terrorist Joey wanted me to loosen my rule to see what the party held for him. He had hoped they would serve hunger. No, Joey, they served pepperoni pizza, and the teen boys in attendance did what teen boys do...*eat*. Eat a lot!

I stood inside the family's kitchen making small talk as I watched and observed at drop off time. I explained that Brother had already eaten, although he could have more if he liked. Of course, I knew such would take an act of God. Nonetheless, I left that afternoon and hoped against hope that this day would be different. A few hours later, my clock told me it was snack time, so his younger brother and I came to pick him up just as they were cutting the cake. The birthday boy's father had dished out nice portions complete with ice cream for everyone. Progress was evident when I saw Brother eating a small single scoop of ice cream. The father indicated it had taken some prodding. The ice cream compliance was good, but not sufficient. I told Brother to have a slice of cake as well, but that we could take it in the car since we had to leave. Brother's gaze and stance then became brutal. He loathed me and his body language said so. The friend's father and mother jokingly encouraged him to take a large slice; of course, not even in their wildest nightmares could they have guessed he was battling anorexia. He was weight-managed so he appeared *normal*, but chaos ensued inside him. This was forced weight management. So I took the slice on a plate, said our thanks, and exited to the safety and solitude of our car.

Brother was angry and had a very hard time consuming that cake. He was upset and complained that it was "excessive" and unreasonable of me to have him eat it. The cake was not the target here. His brain's desire to avoid the cake was the target. Sometimes tough love comes in the form of birthday cake...with icing.

> ***TIP #16:*** *Consider your child's spiritual needs. Prayer is powerful intervention. Fight this illness medically, emotionally, mentally, and spiritually. Get spiritual counsel and guidance from spiritual leaders you trust. The Bible being the utmost authority against refuting the otherworldly stranglehold.*

Pain of mind is worse than pain of body.

— Publilius Syrus

CHAPTER 17

UNDERCURRENT OF PAIN

An interesting thing began to happen as Brother's weight came back on...his emotional intensity increased. In the initial stages, he appeared to be a numb shell, moderately compliant. The main emotion he expressed was indifference, as if he didn't have the energy to fight and he knew he needed help, but he couldn't reach out for it. Then he started to bargain, complain, and object, but this behavior was passive and manageable.

Then when he started to receive nourishment and physically recover, I began to discover his negative thoughts and feelings had another outlet! As the pounds came back, his feelings of being fat increased with an intensity hard to describe. I understand it this way: When he was able to control his food, he could control his feelings. Now he had no control over his eating, so his feelings came out in anger, rage, and anxiety. I had to restructure my expectations of him because the compliant and well-behaved kid who at the age of two never experienced *terrible twos* and wouldn't hurt a fly, was now a raging, unpredictable explosion of emotions 24/7. I won't belabor the point with episode after episode, but simply condense several months here into a summary.

One such event happened at a church Bible study. The Bible study groups are designed around eating, fellowship, and sharing of prayers and praise in a small group format.

Read that again—*eating*! See, everything revolves around eating: holidays, weekend activities, school events, social parties, family gatherings, even church! This is the American way.

As a family, we had been attending Bible study weekly until Brother became ill; then due to the extensive time commitment in the feeding process, we had been unable to attend for many weeks. Nonetheless, we had tried to attend the previous week. I had driven the thirty minutes from home to the study location, only to have Brother break down, crying and screaming over his perceived fatness, and being unable even to get out of the car. So we drove home.

On October 27, I tried again, and we made it successfully through the first half hour. I watched Brother's body language like a hawk and began to notice him crumpling. Literally. Soon he was on the ground of the hosts' home, rolling and grabbing his torso while tears threatened to spill from his eyes.

The rest of the group members were socializing and preparing plates for the meal. I had gathered plates for my children and sat down with them, ready to convince Brother to join me, when I noticed his posture. We made eye contact and he began moaning. Moaning in an animalistic way. I walked over to him and whispered that small children were around so he needed to compose himself. He moaned louder and grabbed his stomach harder. I gathered him up quickly by the arm and walked outside with him, bracing him so he wouldn't fall on the ground. We made it only to the sidewalk before the episode escalated quickly and dramatically. I stood there in confusion and surprise as my child—who by all objective measures appears to be blessed with what society deems as an attractive and desirable physique—threw himself on the ground, grasped handfuls of grass, screamed and yelled, and grabbed his skin until red marks and welts appeared on his stomach. He screamed over and over that he hated himself.

Then he lashed out at me in anger, kicking my shins and clawing my arm as I tried to intervene. He embodied living, moving angst! If he had to eat, then he had to feel, and feeling was so deep and painful that it was expressed in this manner. His internal pain didn't end on the sidewalk. I looked around, frankly afraid the police would be called. Then I gathered him up as best I could as soon as he became momentarily calm, and I walked him to the car. We left and drove home, but Terrorist Joey wasn't through. Brother cried and yelled most of the drive home, and when we arrived, he told me he was sorry, that he was a horrible person, and he spewed a list of self-criticism that was lie after lie after lie. Self-condemning and berating bullying was occurring all in his own head. I counteracted with loving statements and truth until he finally gave up the fight, and emotionally and physically spent, he went to bed.

In addition to no mirrors, no sunglasses, no banded waist clothing, no privacy, no vomiting, no purging, no napkins, no shoes, and no sanity, our home also became a *no sorry* zone. "Sorry" was a banned five letter word. I know most parents pull out their hair trying to teach their children to use this word, but with anorexia comes a high level of self-loathing and self-degradation that is extreme and constant. I coached Brother to say something positive rather than "I'm sorry," which usually led to "I'm a horrible person," "I'm stupid," or "I'm bad." He was none of those things, and even the behaviors he was "sorry" for were truly things he had little or no control over at this time in his life. His brain was a blend of misfiring neurons and emotional haywire. I blamed Terrorist Joey for this chaos, not Brother. I blamed malnourishment for this dysfunction, not my son. Despite constant redirecting on my part, he could not say anything positive about himself or acknowledge any positive self-worth. I hated that he felt that way. Since he had been conceived and first kicked in my womb, I had felt and known his worth and value. My motherhood objective was to raise him to know it himself and to feel it deeply. I felt I had failed.

Realizing the depth of his despair and the anguish of his body and mind, I wanted to help him re-establish his emotional language capacity. With his mind compromised by the effects of malnourishment, he had lost his ability to express emotions verbally. It was as if all he felt was *FAT*. Certainly, all he could identify with was the feeling of being fat. Just as he had reported losing taste preferences while hospitalized, now I realized he had lost his ability to express any range of emotions. One tool I used to encourage his verbal expression was miniature action figures called *emotes.*

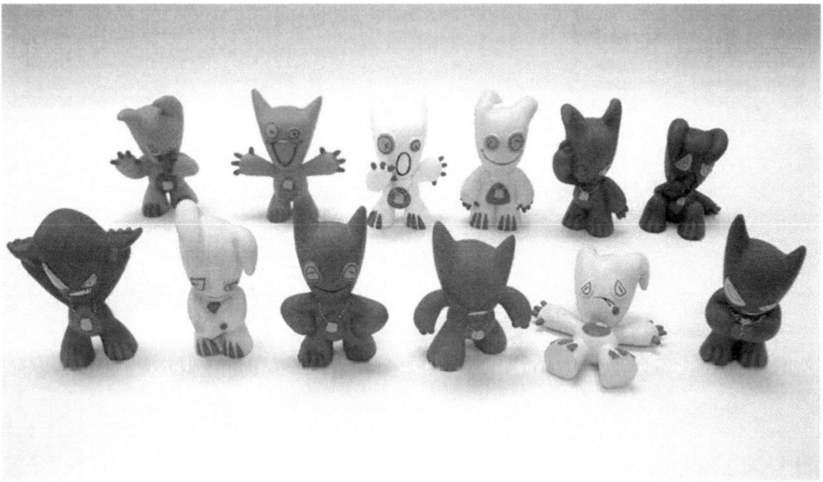

These figures are only two inches tall and one inch deep, but they reach the crevices of the heart and mind. They signify anger, rage, disgust, sadness, exhaustion, insecurity, mischief, confusion, dejection, rejection, love, and happiness. They express what words at times cannot. A language of emotion was needed for Brother to maneuver the muck. Prior to his starvation experience, he had been a communicative child, actually linguistically advanced and highly articulate.

Not so anymore. He could not hold a typical give and take dialogue, much less express his internal world in normal expressions of feelings. It was as if his pain were so deep and raw that it only knew the language of outbursts and excessive motor movements. The pain had no words. My goal was to give him words. These creatures were called to the task. I kept them in my car, and as we drove like maniacs from appointment to appointment to find answers and grasp at healing, I made this a family activity and would ask my children to "find the emote" each could identify with in the moment or the one that represented how he felt earlier that day at school. We practiced. And tried. And tried some more. Brother's response was always that he felt "fat," but with gentle coaching, he would branch out into the realm of actual emotions—yet always in the mad/sad/frustrated/furious continuum. Practicing this with his younger brother seemed to provide helpful role modeling for him to emulate as my youngest son took the lead. In fact, his younger brother provided a positive support and example to Brother in all stages of his recovery by allowing a contrast of normal behavior/thoughts/moods to the inner prison walls erected by Terrorist Joey. One day as we did this emote practice, Brother began crying and said a couple of his classmates had mistaken him for another student—and that student was fat! Well, at least fat according to the assessment of my son and his sidekick Joey! Then he spiraled into believing their comparison clearly meant he was fat and the whole school thought so. He cried and grabbed at his waistline, so to redirect him, I challenged his thoughts by providing alternate explanations (they shared the same ethnicity and hairstyle, etc) and helped him identify the feeling those thoughts caused—insecurity, judgment, fear, etc. It helped some. Eventually, as time lapsed, this became an expected ritual and perhaps somewhat enjoyed. Even when the answer was "I don't know" or I was given a blank glaring stare...Brother was holding the figure, examining the features, and getting the message that *feeling* was normal. Feeling was okay. In fact, he had to *feel* to *heal*. It was a requirement.

> ***TIP #17:*** *Be prepared for emotional angst. When re-feeding occurs, the child will experience increased anxiety. Remind yourself that this means progress is happening! Help your child expand his or her emotional vocabulary to assist him or her with working through this. The eating disorder has likely provided a mechanism for the child to avoid painful feelings. Rather than aligning with this avoidance, assist the child in learning how to express and manage the real internal pain.*

Feelings are much like waves; we can't stop them
from coming but we can choose which one to surf.

— Jonatan Mårtensson

CHAPTER 18

WEIGHTLESS IN WATER

Something about the water beckoned to Brother. Something about the waves appealed to him and calmed him. This was evident to me and to everyone who observed him closely and knew him well. He liked surfing when he left Oahu to visit his dad. But he was obsessed with surfing now. The shift was one of degree and intensity. In some ways, surfing seemed to be a transitional comfort object, much like young children's blankies help them feel safe and secure. My heart was attuned to this in the hospital. It was all he could communicate. The only thing he wanted and was reaching for. How much of this appeal reflected a passion worth living for, and how much of it was him saying he wanted to go home, I wasn't sure.

He wanted to be in Hawaii and along with that he wanted to be in the water. He asked to surf daily. He begged. He had zero energy and we had zero free time, yet the water held promise. Power. When being cared for by Angel Kirsten, the boys often went surfing with her family. She explained to me on several concerning occasions that Brother was incredibly weak, yet he refused to get out of the water. He would want to stay in long past an adequate time, so Heath, her husband, would have to paddle out to retrieve him, and with authority, explain it was time to stop. Brother even approached me one night, surfboard in hand, and out of anger and frustration, threatened to run away and surf alone.

Brother's interest was irrational. It felt pressured. It was positive in the sense that he cared about something. But scary in the sense that he seemed overtaken by it.

I believe water is healing. Water is a life-giving source. Water is a sustaining energy and...it is weightless. The body feels weightless at least. Brother admitted to me at one point that this weightless feeling was true for him, and he "didn't think about *it* (his weight) out there." I think it simplistic to view the pull of the waves as having only one variable; nonetheless, this gravity factor was clearly part of the equation.

We pulled into Ali'i Beach Park to join some friends in watching the Menehune Surf Competition. The boys and I were excited to be enjoying some time on the beach under the warm rays of Hawaii's sun. Even Brother perked up at the prospect of a surfing event. We had a full day planned that involved taking in this competition and then joining an even wider group of church friends for a potluck and praise night at a nearby member's home.

Outings were interesting because they involved some break in our routine, yet they involved the added hassle of preparing and packing all the right amounts and types of food to meet Brother's meal plan caloric guidelines. This day stands out for me because it was when I realized the full extent of paranoia in my son's mind. We plopped our things on the sand and watched the kids put their soul into the sport and catch some impressive three-foot Hawaiian style waves (which equates to five feet or so in mainland measuring). Brother watched in jealous anticipation of his own turn to face the swell. After the competition ended, he begged to go in, and, because of the size of the swell in comparison to his strength at the time, I compromised by allowing him to body board closer to the beach.

He grumbled but conceded and entered the water. He played for quite a while with some of the other children we had met up with, and I had to wave him back in for his snack time since we were keeping with the regimen of six eating times daily. The rule I adopted per his inpatient psychiatrist's instruction was *energy in before energy out*, so this meant lunch before the beach and snack during. This day, like most others, he complained about the quantity and type of food offered. He tried to bargain for fruits and vegetables and was appalled when I required that he eat an energy bar! Oh my, the fat content. Precisely the point, my dear.

I had leverage to use, though, and my rule was if he didn't eat the food I required him to eat, then he couldn't surf or swim because that activity was his current currency. He went along with it and was able to finish an overall successful beach afternoon.

Leaving, though, proved troubling. He climbed into the back of the car with his younger sibling and, because changing in public was overwhelming for him, I handed him his clothes and suggested he change in the back seat. Having adopted some of the local ways of beach lifestyle, we had done this frequently and without hiccup in our previous life, without Terrorist Joey leached onto his brain. Brother started to change, but without looking behind me, I could sense he was having a hard time. His breathing changed. His voice changed, and I felt movement in the vehicle. He screamed "See, Mom! I am fatter than I was before!" and began to cry and moan hysterically. I believe this was connected to his feeling the car shift slightly as he maneuvered into his clothing in a tight, restrictive space. I made the instant decision to drive home and not worry about him changing or even proceeding to the evening's activities. It wasn't worth it and I told him so. I would rather he changed in the privacy of his own bedroom than we continue with our plans at his expense.

He pleaded with me to go on to the event and begged that he wanted to be there. I was appreciative of his growing social interest and saw this as a good sign, but at the same time, I was highly discouraged that such a small task as changing his clothes had triggered him. It seemed no matter what we did, the fat feeling could come out in full debilitating force. As he continued to struggle, I matched his intensity with numerous comments about just going home, but he remained insistent and became angrier and angrier. After a few long moments had passed, I told him he *must* manage his anger. I needed him to use deep breathing or positive thinking and just calm down. When he said he couldn't, out of exasperation, I told him to get out of the car and run around the park—as a release.

The particular beach park we were at had a large grassy area near the parking lot where we were. Brother hesitated and voiced his concern that people were watching. He pointed to a group of four or five teenagers loitering at a picnic table, who indeed were watching the obvious scene now unfolding outside of the car.

Brother whispered, "Mom, they think I am fat, and they will see me run." Yet he clearly wanted to run; the idea of physically releasing his anger was really appealing to him. I countered with, "No, they don't, and who cares?" He would likely never see these kids again, and he needed to run or find another way to calm down or we were going home. "And besides," I added, trying to lessen their credibility, "they are smoking, so who cares what they think?" He was paranoid about what they thought, and in his defense, they did keep staring.

I explained that he was drawing their attention because of his strange behavior, not his waistline! He seemed to accept this and started out with a burst of speed. He made it about thirty yards before he grabbed his side and looked back at me with an expression of frustration and discouragement. I encouraged him on, waving my hands forward. I saw him progress another thirty or forty yards before he fell to the ground in anger, grabbing at the grass and yelling at himself, while writhing like an animal in pain.

"Now, it's become an official scene," I thought.

Somehow, he managed to compose himself and run another short distance, only to repeat the same scenario. Eventually, he managed the full 100 or so yard circle; then panting, he ran up to me with tears and declarations about his failings and fatness. I asked him whether he was ready to go and explained that he had accomplished something hard, despite his thoughts and feelings. I held up a towel and asked him to complete his clothing change under the expanded space outside the confines of the car, which he did. Thankfully.

We drove to the prayer gathering. I questioned myself and fought back the urge to go home anyway because I knew we had another battle on the horizon, the potluck awaiting us. Picture eighty people gathered in a 900-square foot home with some additional garage and outdoor space. It was a hospitable and welcoming environment with lots of loving hugs and caring people, but for me, it was a formidable battle to ensure Brother eat, with people in his midst, and friends now competing for his attention.

I actually let him have some choices in filling his plate, and when he stopped with too little, I just added more. Another shift happened during dessert, though, and Brother's score inched further away from defeat. I explained he had to pick one dessert among the smorgasbord of options, from cake to Jell-O and cookies galore. He reached in, and to my heart's delight, he chose the largest, gooiest M&M cookie on display.

Yes! Were my eyes betraying me? He initiated that! Maybe it was to appease me because he would have had to have substantial dessert regardless. Dare I wonder—could it be that he *wanted* that cookie? Regardless of intent, I tasted a bite of victory in that moment.

Most parents recall the first day their little one sat up, then crawled over, tried solids for the first time, and even took his or her first steps. As the child ages, the events morph into the first day at school, first time driving, and first date. Parenting can be experienced as a series of *firsts*. Since Terrorist Joey had invaded, our *firsts* had changed. The time markers became first time he drank water, first time he ate, first time he made eye contact, first time he sweated, first time he took his jacket off, first time he initiated food intake, first time he wore shoes, first time he leaned back in a chair, first time he made a friend, and so on.

November 4 was the first time he had a good morning. He ate breakfast that morning with his little brother and the whole experience was noticeably different. It was positive. The two boys bantered and laughed together again. They traded stories and smiles. There was a perceptible aura shift. Had I symbolically licked my finger and held it in the air to gauge the emotional wind trajectory, it would have surely shown a shift in direction.

> ***TIP #18:*** *"Energy in before energy out," regardless of your daily activities. Build this mantra into everyday experiences and do not make exceptions even when the schedule is busy and you have to alter plans accordingly. The gain is greater than the loss.*

Listen to what you know instead of what you fear.

— Richard Bach

CHAPTER 19

WHEN THE HEALERS WOUND

Veterans Day, 2013, brought something a military connected family should not have to deal with. Severe unprofessionalism and questionable ethical treatment from the very team I had leaned on to support and guide my family through these dark days. I had the day off and was catching up on chores, cleaning, laundry, and emails. Then I read an email from Brother's nutritionist that made my blood boil. It was a bill for $4,000 dollars.

Paid. From my charge card. Already processed and paid from a credit card number she had asked for during intake, with the explanation that it was a standard paperwork requirement. There was no authorization for these charges.

A couple of weeks earlier, some discontent had begun brewing with Brother's treatment team, specifically his psychiatrist and nutritionist duo. The nutritionist had been highly recommended as an expert on anorexia with years of experience, but she would only treat clients who also agreed to work with the psychiatrist in her complex. For that reason, I had fought hard to find a way for my child's insurance carrier to authorize care with this team. It had been no simple task. I had made the initial phone call to the nutritionist while watching my child, just out of earshot, during the tense trip home in August. I had been told at the time, "Your insurance never has approved me before, but I do accept that carrier if you can get them to." She also exuded confidence and stated that nearly all of her patients recovered and did so without inpatient treatment. As a desperate mother, that was all I needed to hear! If no one had ever gotten approval for this specialty care through my child's insurance carrier previously, then I was going to do all I could to make Brother the first.

My plan was simple—to come prepared to every medical appointment armed with the specific provider's name and contact information and the desperate request of a parent in distress to have the best fighting chance for my son. I wanted someone who understood anorexia because I sure didn't! I needed someone who had experience treating boys with this condition, and she had informed me that she was currently treating three other young boys, which is highly, *highly* unusual!

When I met with Brother's primary care manager, I made this referral request. She submitted it for me. When I met with his military adolescent medicine doctor, I made the same request. He submitted if for me. When I met with his military psychiatrist, I made the same request. She submitted it for me. Somewhere in this chain of requests and referrals, I received a document in the mail, stating in plain English that my son was approved to meet with the aforementioned nutritionist for a total of fifty-two sessions.

Happy tears flowed when I got this news! No more than five minutes later, I had set up an appointment for my son to initiate treatment with her early in the second week of our arrival back on island. We had been seeing her three to four times weekly ever since under the confidence of this preauthorization. The frequency of Brother's appointments was due to individual sessions combined with group meals twice a week. This was our care routine (in additional to medical appointments) until November 1.

I had been noticing marked improvement in my child's eating compliance and was acknowledging that at a pace of four-plus a week appointments, he had gained the weight asked of him, eaten what was put on his plate, and complied with the nutritional expectations to a degree that was worth rewarding. He had been weight restored for a couple of weeks without shifting backwards, yet despite this, I was being told he needed to pack on more weight. This confused me.

I was told his weight was a "moving target" and we needed to continue weight increase because he would continue growing in height through his thirteenth year and beyond. This reasoning seemed abstract to me. I desperately wanted him to continue progressing and not regress, which was the latent threat, yet I was terrified of the anxiety he was experiencing along with the weight gain, so I began to worry about overfeeding him! Standing on a scale confirmed he was in the right zone for his age and height; therefore, I questioned this approach going forward. I had fully and wholly *bought in* up until this point, but I wasn't sure I was mentally or emotionally able to continue buying in to the plan unless I believed it was medically and nutritionally necessary and in his best interest.

When the weight expectation increased, I felt uneasy and asked a lot of questions. My uncertainty grew when I was told, "You have never raised a teenage boy so you can't understand the eating patterns of teenage boys from experience." The nutritionist thought she *knew best* since she had parented teenage boys and knew what *they* ate. Up to this point, I had agreed wholeheartedly with this woman and the direction she had given me. However, I was the expert on my child—not a stranger, regardless of the letters behind her name—and I was able to distinguish patterns that predated his illness, and I told her so.

For instance, he had a couple of vomiting incidents during group meals when potatoes were the expected cuisine. Brother hates potatoes! He has always hated potatoes...and tomatoes. In fact, the first time he had ever eaten a bite of tomato, he had vomited! For me this taste preference was actually positive and signaled a return to a somewhat healthy appetite and tastebuds. When he was back home for the first couple of months, I had been shocked at his complete disinterest in the food on his plate compared to his old pre-summer preferences. After falling ill, he ate everything he was given with the same facial expressions, pace, and reaction... none. Nil. Nada. He seemed strangely indifferent to food, and perhaps, as he had told the social worker in the hospital, it all *was* gross to him, and he ate it all impassively as his watch guard expected.

Maybe one can truly lose tastebuds with this illness. The nutritionist had recommend I feed him a variety of things that involved heavy carbohydrates. One evening, despite my misgivings, I presented him with a large baked potato with cheese and sour cream, large chicken breast, vegetable, and glass of milk. Most of the meal choices were typical for him, but the potato, *oh, my*, his previous self would never have eaten that in a million years, at least not without a fight. Yet there he sat, and without an ounce of protest, he ate every bite. No verbal or nonverbal indication of taste dislike. It was shocking to me then, and shocking to me even now because his taste preferences did end up gradually returning.

During late October, Brother had mentioned several times that despite alerting his nutritionist to this specific food aversion, he was being required to eat potato and tomato dishes. This made it doubly hard for him to attend group and try to meet the expectations there. Still he would eat those dishes because he knew Ensure was the only alternative; nonetheless, a couple of times those foods fought their way back up his throat. This situation was scary because bulimia was a high risk. Binging and purging behaviors lurked around every corner, and Brother's providers and I were hyper-attuned to them.

When he would vomit up these foods, his nutritionist saw defiance; I saw a glimpse of the real Brother!

Because of these incidents and other child-focused reasons, my son wanted to cut back on his group meals. He was vocal about it and voiced his irrational fear that he would "*always* be in group" and "*never* get to leave," and he would break down in tears during these talks. My instinct as a parent was to affirm his progress by listening to him and responding in kind. The challenge, however, was to distinguish Terrorist Joey's voice from my son's. Terrorist Joey wanted Brother to evade treatment and the enforcement of healthy eating patterns. My son, however, just wanted some break in the routine and some normalcy in his world, such as actual homework time and some personal time in the evening. Dare we even think it?

These desires were positive signs in my mind; they resonated with his old self and how he spent his time historically, but I received a large amount of kickback when I voiced my thoughts to his provider. I was told in a very condescending and uncompassionate manner that the recommendation was for two group meals a week, and Brother was not ready to decrease these sessions. She told me she would tell me when he was ready and she did not present it as an option. Her message felt confrontational, and I began to notice a visceral reaction in my body: my heart rate quickened, my muscles tensed, my throat felt tight, and I wanted to leave. I felt attacked and disregarded! My opinion was being treated as irrelevant. I responded that I respected her opinion and recommendation and I would think it over. Yet I left with a very uneasy feeling.

As the next Tuesday group meal day rolled around, we ended up having a very stressful after school experience, so I decided as the parent in charge to keep Brother home and get caught up on life in general. I sent his nutritionist a quick message that he would not be attending and received a curt response that he would be missing two group meals then, due to the next meeting being Halloween. Well, honestly, had I realized that earlier, I would have had him go; however, we were now elbows deep into other commitments, so I apologized for the late notice but stuck with my decision. Had I believed that his attendance was critical for his health, I would have dropped everything and complied, as I had countless times before, but instead, I followed my instinct. I truly wanted what was in my child's best interest, but also not to be at the whim, preconceived notion, or demand of someone else—even a professional.
I had to listen to my own lucid head and be Brother's best advocate. Recall earlier that the professionals at the hospital on the

mainland wanted him in residential care for months, but I had chosen to bring him to this team for outpatient care to provide him with the comfort and safety zone of his own home instead. It was an understandable medical recommendation, yet bringing him home certainly seemed to have been the right choice up until now, and he was responding noticeably to the treatment he was receiving. We ended up missing both group meals that week; once due to parental choice, and the second time because of the Halloween holiday.

It was interesting how nervous I was walking into the nutritionist's office for Brother's scheduled individual session the next week. My heart was racing, I had sweaty palms, and I felt like a kid who had just been sent to the principal's office! She opened her door and called Brother in for his blind weigh in. I heard her question in an accusatory tone, "Why weren't you at group last Tuesday?" My blood began to boil. This had been my decision, not his! And she knew that. He was being drawn into adult matters, and I was outraged. She weighed him and he exited while I was tense as could be, holding back my mama bear.

When the nutritionist called me back into her office, I prepared myself for a mental beat down, which was crazy since I was supposed to be there to get support and help! I took some deep breaths and realized I was going to have to put nice girl aside and be very direct and assertive. I sat down in her office while Brother waited outside. The nutritionist asked me pointedly why I had not brought my son to the previous group eating meal. I explained my reasoning, as I had when I cancelled. I also explained my thoughts regarding going forward in treatment. I assured her that he was receiving benefit from the group meals and I intended to have him continue. I also shared the constraints on our time as a single parent household mixed in with my uncertainty about the treatment plan going forward and reticence to check a proverbial box unless I was convinced of the *why*.

She informed me that she was the expert and her treatment protocol was to attend three sessions weekly, two of them at group. She explained that this was the only option. I was aghast. *Excuse me; was this in writing?* I wanted to scream. My understanding up to this point was that the group meal was *offered* twice weekly, not mandatory. She leaned in dangerously close to my personal space, looked at me like I was a stupid kindergartner, and stated in a solemn tone, "This is going to sound threatening, but I assure you it is not." She continued. "If you continue to be non-compliant with my treatment prescription, I am sure that (insert psychiatrist name) will find out when we have our case meetings and she will refuse to work with your son. She is known for doing that."

Whoa. What just happened! I had been threatened—told to bring him and shut up, in no lesser terms. My body was shaking. She then asked whether Brother would be coming to group on Tuesday. My mind reeled and I informed her I would get back to her after thinking the matter through. I felt put on the spot and pushed into a corner. What was directly stated to be nonthreatening was in fact a veiled threat that felt highly coercive. Again, for a second week in a row, I left that provider's office visibly and emotionally shaken.

The confusion intensified when I received a text from this provider stating that my son's insurance carrier had denied her billing attempt, so I would have to discuss details with her at our next scheduled session. This was a bombshell. Despite some previous back and forth about this issue, and even with insurance preauthorization, received and acknowledged by myself and this provider, concerns remained about billing issues. In fact, this provider had been asking me (as a mental health clinician) how to do her billing! I had called the insurance company to try to solve this problem myself, and I had been told the nutritionist was not currently an active provider and had expired status. In addition, she was coding her profession in a manner that was an unacceptable billable entity for reimbursement. I relayed this information to the nutritionist and requested she fix these areas if possible and resubmit the bill through the proper channels as reflected by the following email:

> Wednesday 11/06/2013
>
> Good morning (name):
>
> Did you get my text regarding ________ conversation

with me and the billing issues? Please advise if there are areas that can be corrected on your end and an expected timeframe? In the light of this very ominous financial stress, I am wanting to know your recommendation for cutting back as I cannot maintain 3 billings per week without this getting resolved. I will be following up with ________ and submitting appeals if necessary, but they advised the two corrections I sent you, and hopefully, we can get back to an informed decision with the billing issue.

For the immediate short term, since (Brother) will be attending group this Thurs, I would like to cancel our Thurs 3pm individual session, and let me know if Monday's 9am with Dr. (name omitted) includes your services as well for a team meeting. Thank you!

My name

The email above was to the *nutritionist*, yet the very next morning, I awoke to the following email from the *psychiatrist*:

Thursday 11/07/2013

Hi (addressed to me),

I wanted to make sure you understand my policy con-

> cerning treatment of eating disorders. Because of the medical seriousness of eating disorders and the high death rate, I do not treat patients with eating disorder unless they are willing to follow all medical and nutritional appointment recommendations, including all appointments (nutritionist name) recommended. Please let me know what you decide to do in terms of following (nutritionist) treatment recommendations. I understand the financial burden you described below, but the death rate is too high in eating disorders for me to take any chances. If you choose not to follow her recommendations, I can provide you with the names of other psychiatrists that (Brother) can follow-up with, or he can be followed at Tripler again. Thank you.
>
> Sincerely, (Name omitted) M.D.

I felt ill. And this wasn't about the money. This was unwarranted. I had only missed one appointment and had given cancellation notice. I debated whether or not to send Brother to group that night. I was actually beginning to sense great hostility and anger from his nutritionist and manipulation through the psychiatrist, and I actually feared retaliation toward my son! I was in a bind, though, because I had told my son earlier that week that he had to go. I was stuck between conceding to Terrorist Joey's wish for him to skip, needing to enforce my authority as the parent, and fearing for my son's experience that night.

And this person was supposed to be a *helping* professional. It was absurd! The clock was ticking and the hour looming, so I decided to send Brother to group. My stomach was in knots the entire time. I felt real terror when my son called from his cell phone partway through the first group hour. It rang once, but before I could answer, it had stopped. I was concerned. He had never tried to call me during group before! He rarely used his phone at all. I called back. It rang and rang with no response. I tried again. Several calls later, I began to worry that she was punishing him in some way and he needed me! That is the level of visceral fear I had reached. I grabbed my keys and told my younger son we were going to find Brother.

The group was eating in town that night...somewhere in a mile radius of the nutritionist's office where the group frequented several restaurants. They alternated between in-office meals and public eating spaces to switch up the expectations and eating demands. I may have looked out of my mind that night; I certainly had unrest in my soul as my youngest and I literally walked restaurant to restaurant, spying into open windows, trying to find Brother. My stomach churned with a nauseated sensation as I grew more and more worried while unable to locate him.

The time neared for the group to end, so we went back to the meeting point in front of her office space and waited there.

Finally, with relief, I saw him. He cried as soon as he entered the car. He said he had tried to reach me because she was making him eat potatoes again. This was not about potatoes. This was about control. Then and there, my heart decided he would not be going back to that environment. I had agonized for twenty-four hours, praying and pondering about what to do before terminating his treatment with this team. He was doing better and I had desperately needed help. It had been working. It was working. I could not imagine not having their expertise and advice. However, I could no longer trust them! They had threatened me, coerced me, and shut down my parental rights. Now they seemed to have taken their discontent out on my son. This was unbelievable and unethical to the *n*th degree. Another decision making crossroad. There was no way I could trust them and their intentions and, therefore, I could not entrust my son to their care. It was incredibly difficult to jump out of the lifeboat that had once pulled us in but it was sinking fast. Difficult but necessary.

The next morning I sent them the following email:

> Friday 11/08/2013
>
> Good morning, Ladies.
>
> I am writing to inform you that (Brother) and I will not be in attendance for the previously scheduled Monday, Nov 11th team meeting session nor any session following. Please cancel that and any reoccurring appointments. As of this date, we will be receiving ser-

vices elsewhere as I have come to the realization that I most definitely need collaboration in my working with his treatment team and have felt everything but that over the last two weeks. I appreciate your interventions over the past few months, but it is time for us to seek healing elsewhere. There is no need for referrals as I have made arrangements.

(Nutritionist), please communicate with ________ regarding billing questions, and I will continue working with them as well to get this resolved.

Thank you,

(My Name)

Bam! Then came Monday when I was charged $4,000 without another word. No more attempts to bill the insurance carrier. No kindness. Just anger and hostility. I believe I was intentionally misled from the start. I believe there were untruths told to convince me to work with this team despite pre-knowledge that insurance would not cover this service. Apparently, my son was a dollar sign for this person. That is the only explanation that makes sense to me. It was horrible. It exacerbated my stress exponentially. But it was still worth it. Brother was making progress. You've got to know when to hold the cards and when to fold 'em. This one I chose to fold.

> ***TIP #19:*** *You can fire your therapist, psychiatrist, or nutritionist. Don't blindly follow medical advice; do your research and ask questions! If you are not getting the help you need with the professionals you are working with, know you have decision-making power, and you truly are your child's best advocate. Do not stop therapy or other services just because the action steps are hard—but do be a discerning consumer and honestly evaluate the care you are receiving.*

Faith to light the darkened sky,
Strength to carry on,
Love to touch and heal the soul,
Hope to grace the dawn.

— Author Unknown

CHAPTER 20

HOPE AFTER FIRING THE HELP

With the cards folding around my professional team, the need arose to find immediate therapy help elsewhere. I felt equipped with the tools and knowledge to continue the nutritional monitoring and expectations, but I was a little leery about trying out my wobbling legs unsupported. We returned to Tripler for nutritional support, and even though the provider there had little experience with this illness, she helped me establish baseline levels of what a child this age and stature should continue absorbing into his cells daily. Recall the three-step process of treatment we were implementing: (1) Refeed, (2) Challenge distorted beliefs about body image and incrementally give eating control back to child, and (3) Address family dynamics and developmental norms.

By this time, my confidence that we were somewhere on the cusp of phase two was rising. Therefore, therapy was extremely important. From working with the psychiatrist/dietician duo, I had some misgivings as to whether or not the psychiatrist would have remained the best fit going forward. Maneuvering the mental health system can be tricky, and I was certain Brother had gotten the help he needed for the re-feeding portion, but his needs had changed, and therefore, the team had to as well. In addition to the mistreatment and unethical dealings, I recalled his psychiatrist telling me that it may be months and possibly years before she could do "therapy" with him. He had a lot of defenses up, and in her opinion, he was not ready to talk about what was happening internally, mentally, emotionally, and family wise. I agreed that his resistance was high, but disagreed that the work toward chipping away at that resistance need be delayed.

My training and experience as a mental health counselor provided me with an alternate view. I have worked with severely dysfunctional children with a myriad of emotional disturbances and had case after case of experiential data suggesting those were precisely the children who needed and could benefit most from therapy. I worried her stance came rather from medical model limitations; no medication = no help. So I began seeking another provider for my son. The psychiatry and psychology professions differ slightly; the former is trained in the medical model (psychiatric medication and emphasis on medical means to restore mental health) versus diagnosis and treatment through talk therapy and assessment measures (psychologist). This line is not rigid and there is overlap and highly qualified help in both realms. Nonetheless, I believe that problems are sometimes unused opportunities. Therefore, this problem with Brother's treatment team became the impetus for taking the next step toward finding the best fit for my son's current struggles.

I was beginning to put pieces together that suggested a male therapist would be helpful. A promising one was found, and we went to an initial session for intake. The therapist was a welcoming person who seemed to share some interests with my son—surfing especially—that suggested Brother might feel comfortable with him eventually. And then, to my disappointment, after Brother left the room, the therapist communicated to me a strong preconceived bias that children with these symptoms are almost always victims of sexual abuse and disclosed a work history that focused predominantly on sexual abuse victims. I understood this concern. Sexual abuse causes an incredible amount of emotional distress. I had read and researched for hours on end. I had talked directly about this concern with all of the treatment professionals to date who specialized in eating disorders.

However, I knew from my reading and inquiry with experts that statistically this is not typically the case. There are many other more likely plausible causative factors. And I am also aware that all providers, including those in mental health, despite good intentions, operate their practices from the bias of their area of expertise and previous work. I wasn't opposed to the exploration of abuse of any nature, but I was leery of a guided exploration that had already determined the cause of onset before the work had begun.

At that point in therapy, I wanted to remain open to analysis of all possible causes until the reason for the mental hijacking could be discovered and the truth known. My clinical opinion was that a host of contributing factors existed. Similarly, my parental instinct believed Brother's situation to be a dangerous concoction of genetic precursor (a family history of anxiety and depression), combined with personality traits (perfectionistic, driven, competitive, high-achieving, conscientious), timing—the merger of childhood and adolescence (developmental stage), identity confusion, troubled family dynamics and the unfortunate opportunity to restrict, having been away from his main home and primary emotional outlet/caregiver. Because this therapist was insistent that sexual abuse was the trigger event, I chose to continue the search elsewhere. I was worried this preconception would be a rabbit trail and potentially damaging.

The ups and downs of getting the right help are hard to capture on paper. Our paths eventually crossed that of a very skillful psychologist who provided immense support to Brother and our family.

> ***TIP #20:*** *Keep knocking on doors until you find a specialist who understands and has expertise with eating disorders. Listen to your child and find a professional who will listen to you. Just do not listen to Terrorist Joey. Treatment needs may change—respond to this. Empathize with the degree of pain your child is experiencing internally.*

Even hundredfold grief is divisible by love.

— Terri Guillemets

CHAPTER 21

LET'S CUT THE TURKEY

Holidays center around food and eating. Even more so when Thanksgiving arrives. This year, I felt immense gratitude that my son was alive and quickening his pace toward health and healing. Angel Kirsten invited us to celebrate the day of Thanks with her family and other island friends. We gratefully accepted. My contribution was a fruit dish, two vegetable hot dishes, and rolls.

We set about that morning preparing these dishes and creating a turkey centerpiece. My heart was light as the significance of this hit me. My son *with anorexia* was helping me prepare each dish! The three of us worked together to prepare the food we would all consume. I could not keep from smiling. When the time came, we gathered at the host's home. It was a beautiful setting and so much thought and great care had gone into the preparations and decorations. Pure joy emanated in the space and on the group's faces.

By this point, I had entrusted Brother with making his own plate. He did so without complaint and willingly ate, yet not the feast I would have chosen for him. I had to encourage him, strongly, to get additional helpings, and there was resistance...yet without a tantrum at least. Jell-O was left untouched. Desserts were left untouched. Cheese was untouched. Stuffing avoided. Turkey and fruit were his go to. It seemed he had accepted that he would eat. Just *what* he would eat and *how much* was still up for debate. After some prompting, we were both mutually satisfied, until the evening wrapped up and dessert remained untouched.

I communicated my expectation that he pick *something*, and eventually, I had to stalk him to the dessert table to get this accomplished. He was upset with me, but he was becoming increasingly social again and wanted to spend time with his friends later—something he knew would be contingent on his cooperation. He begrudgingly complied, and then talk began to spread about a ladies Black Friday shopping marathon. It was starting early this year—on Thanksgiving Eve. While morally objecting, on principle, I went with the flow, just excited to spend some much needed quality girl-time together with friends.

My hesitation was Brother. I hadn't left him alone yet, and I didn't feel right doing so. He would be old enough if you took out consideration of his illness. But with this illness, alone time could mean relapse. A solution proved easy, though, because strangely enough, the middle school children present all wanted to go along! I'm not sure they had any idea what they were signing up for in crowded, congested Honolulu, but nonetheless, the crew of four moms and four youth headed out. I stashed a pear in my purse for good measure! No standing in line would deter snack time!

We waited in Target's line for over an hour, Brother laughing and eating the pear to pacify his mom. He was in good spirits, which was the best part of the outing. He genuinely seemed to be enjoying himself with friends. This would have seemed like a given and obvious *duh* a year ago...but now, it was nothing short of miraculous and a sign of a pendulum shift.

The night went well until we all decided we were hungry and stopped at McDonalds for a quick bite. This wasn't dinner time. This wasn't snack time. This was EXTRA. And Brother resisted BIG TIME. He panicked in the line as his friends ordered Big Macs and sodas and ice cream without reservations. Not my son. He looked at me with large, tearful, pleading eyes and begged...please, Mom, please, Mom, no. NOOOOOO. An immediate calculation went through my head...x slices of turkey plus x pieces of fruit plus x rolls plus x drink and x dessert equals x calories. I knew he was under ratio. Despite the feast today, he had not eaten near what many other attendees had or what would constitute sufficient fullness. I knew despite the vocalization of his mouth, his stomach *had* to be hungry again. So, I decided I *had* to require McD's. We verbally went back and forth in that line, and as we neared the register I was feeling incredibly pressured.

He wanted salad. Only salad. "Okaaay, Mom!" he kept insisting in a pleading tone. I settled for his request for a salad, yet explained quietly that he had to have dressing and he had to have fries or something additional with it. He refused to have a soda. He refused to order more, and he became increasingly agitated. He started yelling at me and causing a scene right there in the Golden Arches' packed house. I ordered anyway with him literally yelling in my ear. This scene had to look strange to everyone observing. I retrieved our order and withdrew far away from our group of friends and outside onto the veranda where Brother could eat in private.

He was fuming. Mad. Irate. Tears spilled from his eyes as he told me, "I hate you." Over and over and over again. My response was, "I love you. I know this is hard, but I love you."

The two security guards eating across the aisle on what was likely their break must have thought I was hurting my son or being mean or something adverse. It looked negative; it felt negative. It was hard. I sat with him as he squeezed his food, scraped off sauce, and intentionally dropped his French fries. I bought him more. Each action required a reaction, and it was a battle of wills on display. I knew Terrorist Joey's agenda—starvation. I knew mine—life. Life with nourishment. It included being able to eat McDonald's when it was the only option you had! Or where the group decided to go. It required being able to pick up a cheeseburger if your life depended on it. It might seem counter-cultural by today's standards. The rest of the world may believe McD's food is bad for you.

True, the nutritional content may be lacking, but that's irrelevant when treating an anorexic! The mental freedom to eat at will was the goal I was after.

It was probably a good hour before Brother completed that meal. The group had long gone off to explore the outlet mall we had arrived at and had dispersed to find the deals they craved. They had thankfully left us alone without question. Brother was immediately remorseful and overly apologetic. He kept repeating over and over that he was stupid, and sorry, and a horrible friend. He cried as we walked, and he said he had missed out. "How long did that take?" he asked with remorse and concern.

I literally supported his frame as we walked, his head on my shoulder. He was weeping, and after I replied, "One hour," he cried even harder and kept repeating the mantra that he was a bad friend, a horrible friend, and *they* must think so. His hypersensitivity to negative evaluation by others was always present in our new normal. He didn't want to miss out! This was far better than not caring! This was a teaching moment, so I capitalized on it. "Do you realize that Terrorist Joey promises you social acceptance and joy if you forego those fries—but the reality is you are miserable? You missed out on an hour of hanging out with your friends all because of a salad *with* dressing instead of *without*. A slight nod suggested he was beginning to realize the cost he was paying and edging toward understanding it wasn't worth it.

Fat fears were the only voice for his internal emotional pain. It was the only perceived control he had. It was all diverted through the *fat* channel. Think about it: it's easier to say, "I'm fat" than say, "I feel unworthy. I feel abandoned. I feel rejected. I feel scared. I feel hurt. I feel unlovable. I feel inadequate. I feel...anything raw or in the deep crevices of the heart."

This lesson hasn't been learned by the majority of adults! We eat—or in his case—reject eating—rather than deal with our emotions. This wasn't about food or fat at all. It was about his self-concept, his lack of self-worth, and his perception of not being "good enough"—all wrongly written on his script since early childhood and enhanced by a summer of prolonged trauma.

The lies were coming into the light and the liar was losing power. We bought sandals that night. His size at the time and one size larger to project the acceptance that growth was good and growth would happen. It was declared so.

TIP #21: *The anorexic's belief he or she is fat is really about self-esteem and self-acceptance. Perfectionism is often an attempt to be "good enough." Validate your child for who he or she is—negate messages that his or her worth is connected to superficial attributes. Children get this message from a myriad of sources. Give voice to the cost this deception is causing in your child's life.*

A person who's going through it, knows pain.
Don't talk to them about being down.
Show them strength and willpower,
they may not know that.

— Gee Linder

CHAPTER 22

THE HIGHER YEAR

It was 2014. The year I hoped would bring complete healing to my son. The year I hoped brought normalcy to my family and our home. The year I counted on kicking Joey to the curb for good! We were invited to celebrate the New Year with friends at our pastor's house. Of course, as with any other American festivity, this gathering centered on food as well as fun.

The pastor's wife was aware of Brother's condition and must have picked up on some of my nerves as the eating commenced. I had positioned myself at the kitchen counter within view of the table where the children had gathered. Brother had wanted to fill his plate with carrots and bare pickings, but I had demanded more. He complied yet wanted to eat out of sight, which made me uncomfortable. He wasn't ready for no accountability just yet, so I monitored.

The pastor came up to us both and jokingly said there were tables set up outside—meant to be used! His wife chirped in that we were content right where we were and would join him outside in a bit. I was grateful to her for that. Too frequently I found I had to explain myself, just be the odd one out, stop abruptly to trail after my son, or be the one to end a conversation brusquely or change the subject because it was going down the trail of doom to topics of diet, fat, weight, bodies, eating, etc.

Brother completed his meal, and off he went, laughing and clamoring with friends. That was different at least and in stark contrast to his summer-fall self! Each time I saw him engage socially, I was relieved. This was normal. I eagerly joined my crowd of peers and enjoyed the adult conversation and games that ensued. Right before midnight, we gathered in the yard to cheer and set off poppers in celebration, and celebrate we did.

We cleaned up, then headed back inside. I got Brother's attention because it was dessert time. He resisted. I insisted. He walked hesitantly around the dessert spread until he gingerly took one small piece of Hawaiian New Year's cake (Chinese: Nian Gao—which means "Higher Year" and is believed to increase your luck in the upcoming year). I required he take two. You see, his friends, of normal appetite and behavior, had been doing the typical holiday *munching* all evening. Not him. And I was onto it. He ate the pieces begrudgingly but quickly, and then he headed toward the bathroom. My mommy intuition began to set off alarms in my head.

For some reason, although Brother had never intentionally thrown up to my knowledge, as I saw him enter the bathroom, my heart began to pound hard and my pulse quickened. "It's nothing, I'm sure," I rationalized. But my feet followed my pounding heart to the bathroom door, and I pressed my ear to it anyway.

What was that sound? Silence, then a strange spitting noise. Silence again, then more strange moisture sounds exiting his mouth. It was not the forceful guttural heaving of vomiting but smaller, more controlled...something...projecting from his mouth. That was enough information for me. I knocked forcefully on the door and demanded, "Let me in." His facial expression registered surprise as he slowly opened the door and defensively said "What!" I didn't want to blame or accuse. I just merely stated what I had heard and asked what he was doing in there. He was dressed and by the sink. He had not been by the toilet; this I could garner by judging the direction of the sounds I had heard. He stammered a bit and said, "Just spitting, Mom." Spitting! Seriously? Spitting sounded like an effort toward calorie expulsion to me.

"Okay, well, no spitting then!" I commanded with definite stress and frustration in my voice. This was now another house rule. "Just don't!" I said with authority and that was that. He understood. Perhaps you may think I overreacted. But I was convinced this was not spitting just to spit. Why in secret? Why after he had just eaten a dreaded dessert? I was dejected that the New Year had started this way.

One positive thing seemed to be a predictable and constant change. He had friends now. Again. He was friendly and developing an ever-growing circle of kids he enjoyed being around. Thursday, December 12, was a day worth remembering. This was the day he told me he had made a friend at school. Prior to this, he had avoided peers and convinced himself this was normal. November was the first month I heard about even remote interest and interaction with schoolmates. Now in January, he and another boy had conspired to spend the day together one Sunday afternoon, and they were working on their respective parents to accept the plan. He wanted to go. I saw this desire as positive, but I was worried, knowing that his friend's family did not know my son well and was not privy to his condition, yet.

With this progress, I reached a parental crossroad where I had to decide whether or not to let him go, and whether to tell the other kid's parents. I chose to let him go and not tell. This was trial and error testing, and I felt we were ready to test his food legs the same way you would let a toddler learn to walk by letting go of the couch! Phase two was in full swing. When I picked Brother up later that evening, the parents told me about all the fun the boys had had, but then they added, "Well, it was strange though... he didn't eat much, even though we stopped for Chinese and had pizza and gelato. But he loves vegetables! We need him around more so our kids will eat their veggies like that. A whole plate of carrots and greens." *Dread.* Interesting how the expectations and roles are reversed for a mind with anorexia. Not only do I have zero problems discouraging sugar and empty calories, I have to coerce him to choose foods beyond those that are raw and just plucked from the earth.

Brother has extreme impulse control! Control that amazes me and frightens me. The issue is not the carrots or the greens or the gelato; it's the thought pattern behind it. It's the motivation that drives the restriction. He's not eating because he *favors* them or has religious and/or health convictions otherwise...rather, he has the fear of getting fat. The fear that consumes him and dictates his fork's every move. That is the problem. I want my child to beat this. I want him to eat what is offered him because it's *just food*. Because he is hungry and he has food to eat and can just eat it! Not because he feels the need to look a certain way or not look a certain way. Not because he feels compelled to subscribe to some socially determined criteria for being *okay*. He is thirteen! I don't want this fear for him now. Not ever. How many of us adults are still fighting this fear? Fear of not being good enough because...fill in the blank—and it's weight-related. How many of us put self-imposed limits on what our stomachs crave because of our fear of gaining weight and then not being deemed *good enough*. By who! This is a crazy mind game with casualties all around.

I continued to support that friendship, but the next Sunday when the boys wanted to hang out outside of my care, I told the other parents about Brother's condition. I told so that Brother had accountability and so Terrorist Joey would not knock on his friends' door for access. Disclosing this was a risk because I did not want his peers to know his condition, but the parents needed to know in order to help monitor. And based on earlier interactions, I believed they would be supportive. Thankfully, they were caring and empathetic and willing to implement whatever I suggested. However, *understanding* is a word that I hesitate to use as a descriptor. They acted surprised and somewhat confused because the child they were getting to know appeared physically healthy to the unsuspecting observer. In fact, others' perceptions was one of the greatest hurdles and frustrations I experienced as a parent trying to help her son overcome this disorder. The professionals I worked with had training and experiences that were amazingly helpful in combating my own confusion. Outside of that, others who understood the subtleties of this condition were rare and few people seemed to *get it*. The general public, our social circle included, was oblivious to the hidden mental traps and fears of an anorexic mind. And because they could not see the inner battle, even the most well-intentioned supporters, even this kind family, would inadvertently say or do things that could cause tantrums or regression. Statements such as "Don't you wish these kids would stop growing up so fast?" or comparative comments such as "I think they can both wear the same size swim shorts if he needs to borrow some; don't you?" I felt like a hyper-vigilant word Nazi everywhere we went! And this made it hard to let Brother go places that didn't involve professional, informed support. Camp was one of those places.

Youth group camp—three words that seem fun when you have a healthy child, but scary when you have had to control or supervise your child's every move for the past six months. Again, to let him go or not to let him go, that was the question. The pitch, a three-day camping adventure over Martin Luther King, Jr. holiday weekend on the shore of Bellows Air Force Beach, on the windward side of Oahu. Friends, fellowship, games, Bible study, and...yep, food. And, let's face it, opportunities for no food. Okay. Deep breathing. *You can do this* (self-talk). And I did. I decided to let go and give Brother a chance to choose food. Without me. My mental consolation was that the camp leaders included Angel Kirsten and her husband Heath, whom I knew and trusted completely and who were already instrumental in his food accountability.

And so he went. And he came back smiling. January 20, 2014, I picked him up as arranged at our pastor's house. We gathered up his things and jumped in the car for the ride home and I asked the question I had been anxiously wondering for three days, "Well, how was camp?" His answer. Brace yourself; I should have. "Mom, I had a sugar rush! I was acting goofy and the kids thought it was funny." "Oh reeeaaallly," I replied and reached around extending a high-five and sporting the biggest smile ever. My youngest son and I made eye contact, grinned, and acknowledged the success in that statement.

Brother went on to share that he had eaten eleven marshmallows during campfire time and his own smile matched mine. I think I just saw Terrorist Joey on the ground with a boot in his mouth, eating dust. Oh the taste of victory was sweet! Really sweet...like marshmallow sweet. And to top it off—I felt a sweet peace from above when I talked to Angel Kirsten afterwards and found out that the camp had a guest speaker address the group and share her testimony of battling bulimia and overcoming it. God works in amazing ways. We just have to trust Him.

Brother's internal change could be witnessed by the evolution of his clothing. From July through October of 2013, athletic wear only, shirts always tucked in, sandals only, and sweatshirt always. Drawstrings a must. By sometime in November he had shed the outer fleece layer and started rolling his pant waist and tucking in his shirts. Sometimes, this *tuck in* process was exaggerated to the point where I had to inform him he had *tucked in* his underwear as well and they were showing! This didn't faze him. He was over-concerned with the waist and under-concerned about the skivvies. Still sandals only. By the second week of December, he was leaving his shirt untucked and wearing shoes! And continuing to avoid the unnecessary constraints of winter gear in a summer climate.

Fast forward to January, 2014. On the sixth day of a truly New Year, Brother told me he wanted to be homeschooled because he looked fat in his school uniform shirts—"but other shirts are better." I focused on the positive and minimized the negative. Emphasis on his acceptance of his body in other shirts. Hallelujah.

Then behold, January 7, he actually took off all layers to the world and slept with his shirt off! Major progress. From multiple layers of clothing to bare skin! This may sound strange, but I was ecstatic to see him on January 8 walk past me headed to bed with only boxer shorts and a grin. His younger brother and I both, recognizing the dramatic change occurring, stopped what we were doing and shared another glance. This meant he accepted himself. Physically at least. He saw that he was *okay*. He was announcing this and letting it be known to his family that he could be okay in his own home with his own body. Even his nine-year-old younger brother noticed this and acknowledged its significance nonverbally. I may have literally raised a fist of triumph in the air that night.

> ***Tip #22:*** *Balance carefully the need to monitor eating disorder behaviors with your child's increasing freedom and control over eating choices. There are no holidays from being a watchdog in your child's life until feelings stop being diverted through the "fat" channel. When this happens, learn to give back eating control, first gradually and then fully, while always mindful of the potential for relapse and being vigilant against any warning signs.*

If you are distressed by anything external,
the pain is not due to the thing itself,
but to your estimate of it; and this you have
the power to revoke at any moment.

– Marcus Aurelius

CHAPTER 23

THE HIJACKER GETS EJECTED

From that day forward, Brother continued climbing the road to healing, and slowly but surely, reclaiming his body and acceptance of it. In fact, after that day, relaxing in boxer briefs became the norm in the comfort zone of his home. He could be himself behind these walls.

Sometime during late February, I noticed meals were fun again. Brother could sit anywhere in the car he wanted. He became interested in completing schoolwork again—and he had the attention span and mental capacity to do so. His grades started to climb. He played with his brother again, true, give-and-take dialogue and playfulness. Eventually he was entrusted with lunch time at school and passed this test with flying colors.

I requested his school keep him on the monitored snack regimen for the rest of the school year, for an extra buffer between him and the feared restrictive urges. It was kind of like leaving a remnant of soldiers behind in case the enemy returns. Life went forward, and with it came a return to more and more normalcy.

Great things happened in 2014.

In March, during Spring Break, my sons and I celebrated recovery. We went to Australia on the adventure of a lifetime to revel in life and all that had been overcome. We did this to honor our clan-like love and to fulfill a promise made to Brother when he was in kindergarten. When Brother was five years old, he was an avid Crocodile Hunter fan and spent hours glued to the Discovery Channel and consuming all media related to reptiles, the ocean, and animal life.

At that point in our life, we were living in Missouri, surrounded by land and more land with no inkling of when our path would cross the ocean. Yet I found myself telling Brother, "When you get older, we will have a mother/son adventure to scuba dive the Great Barrier Reef." He had lit up from ear to ear, and we talked about how amazing that would be. I had no idea how it would ever come to be. Now fast forward eight years, we lived in Hawaii, were both scuba certified, and he had overcome a significant time of adversity. Then, surprisingly and completely unplanned, Angel Ingrid, out of the generosity of her heart, provided us with standby fare to go anywhere Hawaiian Airlines flies. It felt like a gift straight from our Heavenly Father. I was so happy still to have Brother in my world and to deliver on my promise.

Even better yet it was a mother/son/son adventure and both my boys got to be brothers again. As we flew from Hawaii to Australia, I could not keep from watching and noticing Brother. Watching him smile and laugh and say, "Yes" to the stewardess' offer of snacks and accept the drink and consume it without hesitation. I heard him talk about all the things he wanted to see and do. I watched him banter with his brother, while sitting completely comfortably with his back touching the seat and wearing shorts and a T-shirt. He no longer wore the cologne of death.

Flashbacks of our last flight contrasted immensely with this one. If he had picked up a terrorist on his last flight away from home, he was leaving him on this one!

After landing, we explored. We strapped on the oxygen tanks and dove the Great Barrier Reef at Lady Musgrave Island—it was symbolic of the depths of pain he had overcome and the fullness of life he still had to experience. Our family laughed together, camped together, and ate together. It was during this trip that I realized with great joy that Brother chose *soda*. The food restrictions began and ended with soda. The illness began and ended with a flight over the ocean. Not to say there were zero obstacles after that trip. But Terrorist Joey was gone and Brother was back.

Tip #23: *Celebrate progress. Expect triumph over this illness and take a positive stance that victory will happen and your child's life will be restored. Verbalize it and claim it. Your child needs you to be confident about this.*

Genetics make the gun, and cultural and familial environment loads it, but it takes the experience of unbearable emotion to pull the trigger.

— Aimee Liu, *Gaining: The Truth About Life after Eating Disorders*

CHAPTER 24

A DANGEROUS CONCOCTION

Now that we had rid our family of the unwanted hijacker, I wondered with great sadness: How did Terrorist Joey gain access into my son's mind? What caused Brother's anorexia? Why did this happen? As I processed my child's suffering, what his life had been reduced to, and how far he had come to reclaim it—the price he paid (hours and days and weeks and months of starvation and anguish)—you bet I asked why. I am certain you are left wondering the same. Is society to blame? Was this a genetic curse? What does puberty have to do with it? Did something happen to him that summer? Was trauma involved? Does the family structure play a role?

Just as I had taken a holistic approach to targeting and responding to his varying symptoms, so my belief in my child as a multifaceted being with varying influences certainly plays into my analysis of his succumbing to the terror of Joey. My clinical experience has reinforced in my mind that all human behavior has to be examined through more than one lens. *Yes* to all of the above.

Why is a luxury—sometimes, it is never known, and other times, no one ever dares to explore it. It can be counterproductive to fixate on it when the child is literally dying in front of one's eyes. Yet after re-feeding has occurred, and after the child has dealt with distorted thought patterns and worked through body image issues—should we not look at the why? Every case needs to be evaluated on an individual basis and will involve unique circumstances. Yet, just as there are guiding principles on the treatment of this illness, I believe this illness doesn't happen to children haphazardly and without explanation.

The mind and the body are inextricably intertwined. The genetic wiring dances with the experiences of life. There is high probability that something in the environment triggered the food restriction snowballing into the full-blown disorder of anorexia nervosa. This could have been familial, social, cultural, mental, or chemical in nature. With any behavior and thinking gone awry, there is the challenge of *teasing* out the contributing variables. The fact that anorexia occurs mainly in highly industrialized, wealthy countries suggests a socio-cultural contribution to the medical picture. I have already discussed the troubling frequency with which media messages bombard our youth, pointing out what is wrong with them (body image being the main target), and then touting promises of how to fix those flaws. This marketing ploy strikes at the innocent and vulnerable mind, where it is absorbed and assimilated to some degree—and in some minds more than others.

Take a perfectionistic kid who has high-impulse control and the genetic blueprint for strong willpower and then is raised in a culture where he or she hears incessantly how to live life *right*. And this subliminal *right* is defined as a certain look, accomplishment, number, or other superficial barometer of acceptance and value. "Another part of the growth of anorexia may have to do with the growing focus on educating kids about obesity," states Johanna Kandel, founder and director of the Alliance for Eating Disorders Awareness in West Palm Beach, Florida. "There's been so much emphasis on childhood obesity, all these programs to ameliorate the situation and in a way we're actually potentiating eating disorders. That's a very thin line we need to walk and make sure the dialogue is one of a healthy attitude toward food." (12)

To add to this recipe, consider the role of hormones and the developmental stage of puberty. Anorexia often strikes at the intersection of childhood and adolescence or between adolescence and adulthood. These milestones involve surges of hormones that signal changes in many aspects of youths' lives.

> Adolescence is a time of transformation and growth physically, mentally and biologically. This is a time when

> children move towards adulthood, and begin to discover who they are. They become more independent, establish friendships, and their bodies develop. This development is obvious physically, but there is also a large amount of change happening internally, especially in the context of hormone levels. For many, entering into puberty can be a very emotional, stressful, confusing, and frightening time. In addition to the physical and hormonal changes, there are social mechanisms at work. Studies show that when a child hits puberty, his or her brain's socio-emotional system changes and this is seen as an increased concern in being socially accepted. In ecological terms, this is a natural progression into sexual maturity and the social responsibilities that go hand in hand with getting older. As a result, the teenage brain seeks reward from being popular among peers, and behavior is often focused on activities and ways to be more socially accepted. Dieting is one such behavior that teens engage in in the hopes of being socially accepted and dieting may in turn trigger an eating disorder in some individuals who are genetically predisposed.
>
> There are also theories that the hormonal changes as they happen in puberty initiate the activation of genes that predispose individuals to eating disorders. (13)

All of this is a storm brewing underneath the surface, and because anorexia is characterized by distorted thinking, Terrorist Joeys around the globe are slipping in with false promises of making this internal storm stop. I recall Brother's comment to me on that flight over the Pacific to return home. At least some part of him didn't want to grow up. Growing up means embracing the change: body change, expectation change, social pressures, relationship development, separation from attachment figures, individuation, and identity formation. These are tough times!

Erik Erikson is a child development theorist who insisted that "the adolescent's task is to synthesize past, present, and future possibilities into a clearer sense of self." (4) He surmises that the task of "identity versus role confusion" is central to this stage of development and the resolution of this task will be either successful or unsuccessful. When unsuccessful, the child stays stuck emotionally in this tumultuous period. When successful, the child moves on to the next stage of young adulthood: love and work. Youth, therefore, try out different aspects of the self—deciding which fits. This search for the self comes through descriptive labels and self-ascribed roles, usually aligning with their deep emotional need for approval and acceptance. Children decide "I am Goth," "I am a bookworm," "I am smart," "I am a star athlete," "I am the class clown," "I am the pretty one," "I am the ditz," "I am the overweight slob," or "I am the skinny kid." The skinny kid is socially acceptable. Overweight slob is not. If somewhere in this chaotic role assignment, the pursuit of skinny becomes a fixation and the focus of identity formation, the role play can turn tragic.

My understanding of this is both professional and personal. I came close to being anorexic myself. In fact, I remember very well my thought process at age twelve. I have a distinct memory of belonging to a very small class of students in the sixth grade. During this formative time, I was told frequently by peers and adults in my world that I was "skinny." This was stated in approving tones and social acceptance followed. I attended an unusually small private school and roles were easy to obtain and clearly defined. There were literally three students in my class: the troublemaker boy, the fat girl, and the skinny girl. Then my world was disrupted—a new girl was added to the mix. I remember the emotions that news created: fear, jealousy, and anxiety. I was the skinny girl! No one could take that from me—*could they*? Such a possibility caused me great angst. If I were not the skinny girl anymore, what was I? *Who was I?* I had no answers.

Then she showed up to class—skinny girl. Another skinny girl! What would happen? I felt threatened somehow. My body shape by genetics was small framed and average by most standards. Yet my fears of displacement were valid and strong. Strong enough to fuel the distorted thought that "I *had* to be the skinniest girl in sixth grade," and "When I am skinny, I get attention and approval and people will like me more if I lose weight." The fear trumped my hunger pangs and trampled the instinct to respond to food cravings. Those thoughts and feelings motivated my behaviors: I stopped eating for two weeks. And I failed as an anorexic. I started eating again because it was too hard. I diverted my energy to being "pretty enough" and "skinny enough" (rather than the skinniest)—maintaining a shaky enough self-image that I fell prey to people in my adolescence and young adulthood who perpetuated the belief that I was only as good as my body and face. I was vulnerable to this because of the messages I had been given as a child by society and through unmet emotional needs as a girl desperate for her father's approval. I did not know my own worth. I did not feel "good enough."

A sad reality. One that I have overcome and can look back on with insight and sadness. And great relief for the narrow escape I had made from Terrorist Joey. Now, with deep pain, I wondered what this genetic, societal, and familial legacy contributed to my own son's body image struggles. Was the common denominator a genetic code, an age bracket, or the wrong answer written into the soul about our value and inherent worth?

A gender specific complication is worth including into this exploration. Not just "Why did anorexia happen to my child—but why did this happen to my *male* child?" Anorexia rarely strikes those of the male gender. How does a boy establish identity? How does he see himself develop as a man at this stage? Psychologists have embraced numerous theories for understanding this phenomenon, yet a worthy summary is the role of modeling in human behavior. Boys need boys to teach them how to be men. Boys need good men to teach them good character that aligns with the sense of self the child needs to have (even more so, to be egosyntonic, especially for a perfectionistic child). Complicating this identity challenge is the reality that my sons have grown up in a fatherless home. This can happen in homes with emotionally absent as well as physically absent fathers. This concept is pertinent to the complete picture because a mom cannot help a son discover manhood in the way a man can. I fear that Brother fell under the following description: "Boys raised mainly under the supervision of women—Mom, female teachers, female Sunday school teachers, female Cub Scout leaders—often experience insecurity over their identity as men." (14) Brother certainly had some resistance over embracing his growth into manhood. His illness was a complete regression into early childhood in a physical, emotional, and mental sense. It may have indicated a subconscious wish to stay in that state or a wish to avoid the anxiety over becoming a young man, which he had some negative associations with. Manhood, in his experience of the role, did not always equate to strength, loyalty, courage, and protection. This intuitive knowledge conflicted with his internal desire to do things well.

An additional consideration is that Brother likely had the genetic predisposition for this particular illness. When you sit in a room of eating disorder patients gathered for a support group, you realize something rather quickly. These kids share common traits. They are almost all high achievers, driven, intelligent, rule-abiding, conscientious, focused, competitive, perfectionistic, socially accepted, and all around *good* children. One of the emotional and mental challenges a parent deals with when the diagnosis is made is: "This can't be happening to *this particular* child."

Disbelief. Denial. These children seem to have it all together, cope well, and don't make waves. Then bam—they are faced with overcoming the deadliest psychiatric disorder in the diagnostic manual. It has nothing to do with anything being wrong with the child, and it certainly isn't something anorexic sufferers choose. They did not wake up and decide to straddle the chasm of life and death! Their brains were hijacked and they found themselves fighting for their lives—but no personal ownership for the dice landing on *AN* is required here. Neurology is a contributing culprit. In fact, brain imagery advances have been paving the information highway and helping doctors and scientists understand the structure of anorexic brains as compared to healthy brains:

> "It's very rare for me to see a person with anorexia in my office who isn't a straight-A student," Lock says. Even at an early age, people who later develop the eating disorder tend to exert an almost superhuman ability to practice, focus, or study. "They will work and work and work," says Lock. "The problem is they don't know when to stop."
>
> In fact, many scientists think anorexics' brains might be wired for willpower, for good and ill. Using new imaging tools that let scientists watch as a person's mental gears grind through different tasks, researchers are starting to pin down how anorexic brains work overtime. (15)

Every single person walking the face of this planet has a genetic vulnerability of some kind. Perhaps high blood cholesterol runs in the family. Or heart disease or hypothyroidism. Perhaps a child is born with the precursor for schizophrenia or depression. I haven't heard yet of a person, outside of Jesus Christ, who can claim an infallible genome! As a member of his extended family, Brother had genetic traits transferred to him chromosomally at the moment of his conception. He inherited more than hair and eye color. He inherited a greater risk of obsessive and compulsive tendencies which he may have shared with me, as evidenced by my own struggles with these issues when I was a child seeking to control private insecurities and fears. Although never diagnosed or formally treated, my own need for control in an uncontrollable world came out in anxiety laden ways. He inherited an increased risk of anxiety and depressive ailments from his paternal lineage. And he was the recipient of perfectionistic traits from both sides of his grafted family tree. Along with his gender, hand dominance, intelligence, and height potential, these aspects of who Brother was involved gifts as well as time bombs—waiting for the right time to detonate.

I see all of these variables as slices of a pie. Each child could have varying numbers of slices and differing sizes of each. Yet the dangerous recipe is in the combination—and having a trigger event or environment. Perhaps that trigger is never identified. Let's consider the family system as a pie piece. Present in the total anorexic pie for some, not necessarily for all. For Brother, I believe this is the final piece of the puzzle and the key to unraveling his anorexia. And also a necessary part of successfully completing phase three according to family systems theory .

The very title of the three phase treatment approach as described by our psychiatrist/nutritionist treatment team suggested *family matters*. I have explained that although the Maudsley Approach: Family Based Treatment guided my understanding in terms of weight restoration and identity formation challenges, here is where my family counseling training diverts from the Maudsley model. Essentially, I see cause and treatment as different discussions. This is a very delicate topic and one I approach rather tentatively. Just as there is no cookie cutter recipe for treatment of all cases of anorexia, there is no simple cause and effect mold to try to understand the illness' onset. From my reading and understanding of the Maudsley method, the family is seen as the best chance for help and recovery—certainly not the target of blame. And I would concur that, in my experience, the family *is* the best hope a child has to fight the terrorist inside and reclaim his or her head space. It certainly proved true for Brother. And that is the only truth I can speak. Our family's truth—that which I witnessed and experienced.

I emphasize with urgency that the first and foremost agenda when faced with this destructive illness is to treat it. And that treatment must involve family! Family members are the hands that feed and the voices that say "Yes" to food when the sufferer cannot. Moms and dads and brothers and sisters can give love, unconditional support, and care even through barrages of verbal assaults during re-feeding. They can hold, hug, and soothe when the emotional tides of anger and rage flood the brain's synapses. In my opinion, there is no good substitute for a parent's arms or a loving caregiver's support in battling this deadly disorder.

Jacquelyn Ekern, the founder of Eating Disorder Hope, in describing family therapy as an intervention tool, states: "This method of therapy is generally classified according to the types of interaction between family members and accentuates family relationships as an important factor in psychological well-being. A similarity among the different components of family therapy is the belief that encouraging family participation and involvement in solutions is advantageous." (16)

Yes, indeed, the family is an incredible source of healing. Without negating that message—the family can also be a source of pain. Deep, guttural, animalistic pain. I have extensive educational background and training that views the family as a system, so when an identified patient presents with such a clear cut emotional and thought-based diagnosis, it is hard to say with certainty that family dynamics make zero contribution to an illness' development. Nor am I suggesting that across the board, all cases of anorexia and bulimia involve family dysfunction, nor that such causes other forms of disordered eating in general, such as obesity or unspecified eating disorders. To infer so would be inaccurate. I do not mean these words to be a blame game, nor a generalization. Nonetheless, my training in family systems and all of my clinical experience to date suggests that to overlook this variable would be a disservice to some cases where this is an important contributing factor to the illness' cause.

Personally, I can say with 100 percent confidence...something horrible happened to Brother that summer. Countless people have suggested that—professionals and laymen alike. The drastic decline Brother went through emotionally and physically is mind-boggling and suggestive of an emotional whiplash. Maybe the "horrible thing" was the slow starvation itself and nothing more. A near death experience from starvation would be categorized as "traumatic" by any definition of the term. I have directly asked Brother what happened and he becomes tearful and responds that he doesn't know. Maybe he does know and it is too hard to acknowledge even to himself; perhaps he knows and doesn't want me to know, or perhaps he truly doesn't know. There are numerous hypothesis that can be presented. All of them hard to consider. My head and heart have considered each one. Without the benefit of observational evidence at the time of anorexia's onset, I have analyzed and evaluated a host of potential variables and I agree with the general audience.

Something happened. I just think that *something* was not a distinct event as some people might be inclined immediately to suspect. Rather, my fear became that it resulted from an indirect, subconscious absorption of a situation that was toxic.

I understand this situation as being similar to the way cancer may develop. Cancer cells are not new cells introduced into the body; rather, they are the cells that have already gone awry and grow at an abnormal rate rather than dying normally. The American Cancer Society explains:

> Cells become cancer cells because of damage to DNA. DNA is in every cell and directs all its actions. In a normal cell, when DNA gets damaged the cell either repairs the damage or the cell dies. In cancer cells, the damaged DNA isn't repaired, and the cell doesn't die like it should. Instead, this cell goes on making new cells that the body doesn't need. These new cells all have the same damaged DNA as the first cell does. People can inherit damaged DNA, but most DNA damage is caused by mistakes that happen while the normal cell is reproducing or by something in our environment. *Sometimes the cause of the DNA damage is something obvious, like cigarette smoking. But often no clear cause is found* [italics added for emphasis]. (17)

For some cases of cancer, not all, there is a supposed trigger that *sets off* the abnormal cell growth and seems to *turn on* the cancer trajectory when logic suggests that perhaps without this trigger, the switch could have been prevented from flipping. A neuroscience concept is that genes are *self-regulating*, a concept defined by the National Human Genome Research Institute:

> Gene regulation is the process of turning genes on and off. During early development, cells begin to take on specific functions. Gene regulation ensures that the appropriate genes are expressed at the proper times. Gene regulation can also help an organism respond to its environment. Gene regulation is accomplished by a variety of mechanisms including

> chemically modifying genes and using regulatory proteins to turn genes on or off. (18)

This concept applied to Brother's diagnosis of anorexia nervosa is that there was a *trigger environment*, and this contributed to the onset of anorexia and, therefore, to pretend otherwise would perpetuate a cycle of denial and subsequently block off the path to true healing and awareness. Brother expressed this himself in numerous actions and statements as he was recovering. During his healing process, it seemed as if the layer between the conscious mind and the unconscious was peeled back and revealed. There was no "filter" or ability to repress the depths of this pain and awareness. Years of stifled emotions surfaced. The brain's normal defense mechanisms became accessible again after Terrorist Joey's eviction—but in his raw compromised state, his cognizance was expressed in ways his healed mind could not easily access.

Mentally and emotionally, Brother reacted to what I believe was an intuitive relational awareness and internalized family dysfunction pain. His pain had a history and a context. This wasn't just about the impact of social media and puberty. It was the coping mechanism of an emotional hunger that could not be met, and subconsciously found its expression in an experience of physical hunger!

In Brother's descent into despair, I believe he succumbed to the external societal message of inadequacy and internalized it as truth. And this inadequacy message was disastrously combined with a troublesome internal message written on the script of his childhood and experienced in the events of that summer. Would his anorexia switch have turned on without these ingredients?

In fact, the words of Dr. Anita Johnston summarize this most accurately. Dr. Johnston is an expert psychologist in the treatment of eating disorders and founder of 'Ai Pono Hawaii ('Ai—*to eat, nourish* Pono—*with ease, naturally, and in perfect order and wholeness*), writes about her philosophy as it developed in the 1980s as she worked with sufferers of disordered eating at a day in age when very little was known about the *why*:

> What was it about these particular individuals that caused them to face such overwhelming struggles? And why were their struggles getting expressed through food, eating, and body issues? One of the prevailing theories at that time was that eating disorders were caused by trauma. However, although many of the individuals I was seeing indeed had had some traumatic experiences in their lives or had had difficult childhoods, there were many more who came from loving, intact families and had had no significant trauma.
>
> And so, because I am a storyteller, and because as a psychologist I am a trained story listener, I began to listen very closely to their stories, trying to find some clue as to what might be behind or beneath their struggles with food, fat, and dieting.
>
> What I discovered was that these individuals were very much like the outspoken child in the fairytale, The Emperor's New Clothes. They were highly intuitive, emotionally sensitive, and

> seemed to have an innate capacity to perceive subtle realities: they could read between the lines, perceive hypocrisy, see the bigger picture, or sense when things were not okay even when everyone around them said everything was just fine. Unfortunately, when they spoke candidly about their impressions and said, "The Emperor has no clothes," they were either ignored, rejected, ridiculed or, in some cases, abused.
>
> It soon became apparent that the disordered eating functioned as a mechanism to help them cope with their "thin-skinned nature." It enabled them to stuff their truth, quiet their voice, and dim their light so they could fit in. It was the best way they could come up with to distract themselves (and others) from their "differentness," which they interpreted as a flaw and cause for their feelings of alienation. Unfortunately, this adaptive mechanism began to take over their lives, ultimately creating more problems than it solved. (19)

Dr. Anita Johnston has thankfully acknowledged rather than skirted the emotional pain the eating disorder signals to the outside world. The feelings that cause a person to deny basic primal needs have to be included in our understanding of the development of all forms of disordered eating. General knowledge abounds that overeating can sometimes be caused by *emotional eating*. Why, then, should the other side of the eating continuum not be included in such a discussion? Bulimia and anorexia are cries for help and simultaneously a cluster of symptoms that are self-destructive, with the end goal being to look in the mirror and like what one sees, and with weight being the primary external indicator of internal worth. The disconnect the sufferer has with the outside world parallels the numbing involved in substance abuse. Maybe wasting away to nothing and feeling hunger pangs is better than feeling unworthy or inadequate in the anorexic mind. It is abuse of the self, acted out because the self is deemed unacceptable. Maybe for some that message was explicitly demonstrated or stated in abusive ways. *But maybe not?* Maybe instead that message was one of subtleties and just as in "The Emperor's New Clothes," they read between the lines.

So then *what* comprises the *why*? Genetics, brain anatomy, hormones, society, media, culture, gender, age, developmental tasks, trauma, or family dynamics? All of these variables are worth considering when tweezing out the underlying contributing variables on an individualized basis. No cookie cutter equation exists for treatment or for cause. A distinguished psychiatrist, Dr. M. Scott Peck, informs "There is a rule in psychiatry that all significant psychological problems are overdetermined—that is, that they have more than one and usually many different causes, just as plants will often have many roots." (20) In writing this chapter, it is my hope to spark dialogue so that awareness is increased about the forces at play behind the illness. Therefore, treatment can be tailored and targeted to the multifaceted cause through efficacious professional help.

Tip #24: *Don't get stuck in a blame game. Likewise, don't deny family, social-cultural, interpersonal, or neurological dysfunction if it exists. Understand that eating disorders don't develop as simple cause and effect equations—yet at the same time, seek therapy to unravel any emotional hunger that needs to be addressed.*

Breathe deep,
sing loud and sweet,
I am me,
I am unique,
I am magnificent.

— Jonathan Lockwood Huie

CHAPTER 25

A SECOND KIND OF DELIVERY...DELIVERANCE

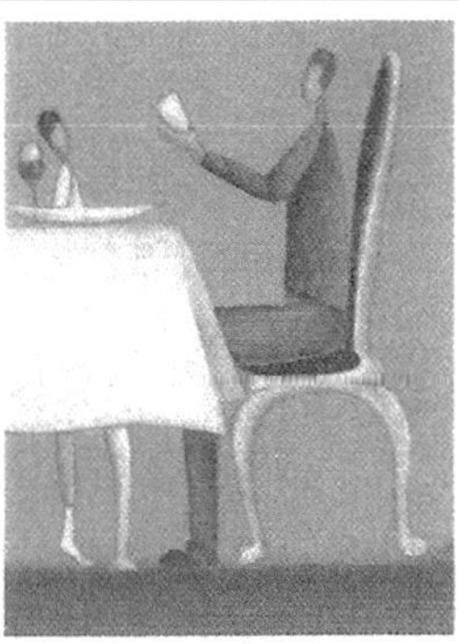

If you could go back and repeat one day of your life, which day would it be and why?

Reprinted with permission.

March 5, 2014. Dinner time. Our family was in a much better place. We were sharing "Food for Talk," which was a tradition in our home. We used recipe-sized cards that provided numerous conversation starters on a wide range of topics. The card pulled from the box this evening was, "If you could go back in time and relive one day, when would it be?" Brother went first. He jokingly but solemnly at the same time said June 7, 1883. June 7 was the serious part—1883 denoted the safe territory of jest. June 7 was the day he left for his dad's! It was the last day I saw my son before his emotional hijacking. This was an indirect way of saying he wished he could go back in time and not get on that plane. Yet by inserting "1883," it seemed to maintain an acceptable response without being disloyal to his dad. He was home and he was recovered. But he was sad he went through the experience at all. With all seriousness, the benefit of hindsight, and no conflicted loyalty, I said my wish would be to redo June 7, 2013, and I would have refused to let him get on that plane. He nodded in appreciation and agreement.

The boy who could not complete the simple math problem of 50 x 3 at the start of the eighth grade, went on to take the eighth grade ACT at the end of the year and received high marks—21 out of 25, and in the English subtest, he scored 100 percent, the highest grade possible. He also completed the Hawaii State Assessment (HSA) and received marks in the excelling range. By spring, he had raised his science grade from 5 percent to 77 percent, and it was still climbing. He was chosen captain of his baseball team, accepted into a preseason high school basketball club, and had been asked to join a second basketball club on the island. When I ran into his school principal in April, she could not believe that this young man was the same person. This external validation aligned with my inner relief and celebration.

Just as the descent into the valley was observable by the physical senses, so was the realization that the valley was behind us. Where my eyes before saw a skeletal frame, the tremble of a shivering body, and odd excessive movements, now my eyes registered a healthy skin tone displaying a frame that was comfortable in its space and eyes that lit up when Brother smiled. My eyes gratefully noted the way he walked in a straight line, no longer zigzagging, and how he moved as if he had a right to be on this planet. Where my nose once smelled decay, it now smelled the blessed gift of sweat and the aroma of food chosen at will. Where my ears once missed the sound of laughter and normal sibling banter, they now heard the blessed sound of boys wrestling and arguing because they both had opinions deemed worthy of being expressed. Where my body once felt the adrenaline of a fight or flight crisis and an indescribable, persistent ache in my heart, I now felt the sweet sensation of giving my son a high-five and a hug, and it being reciprocated. Sometimes the gift of the here and now is realized through the pain of the past.

It had taken nine months for this precious child to develop from a zygote to a fully formed fetus in my womb before birth, now we had essentially experienced a nine-month process of physical rebirth (August-April). He had gone from death's door to fully restored health in this formative time. April, 29, 2014, I realized the child sitting in my living room studying and completing his schoolwork without hindrance—singing, smiling, listening to a new tune on his iPad, and asking for food—was Brother. Truly Brother. Without the remnants of Terrorist Joey. Without a hint of what happened to him the past summer. It was hard to reconcile this person with the individual I walked with through the valley of the shadow of death. These kinds of things could be easily and readily repressed. His eyes were clear with a glint of glee and lightheartedness. He had shed the dark glare of death. He acted as if he had a second chance at living. Like a cancer survivor who can't stop smiling, his joy was palpable. It was a transformation that I have to bear witness to. After a long day of work, I had prepared myself a bowl of cereal and sat down to enjoy its contents, knowing that Brother was busy with the task at hand and would be receiving a snack later. Casually and without hesitation, in response to what must have been true appetite signals in his stomach, he asked me, "Can I have a bowl?" Phase three, Maudsley model, was in full swing.

He had been eating willingly without any complication for a couple of months now. But still, he had just recently risen to the level of initiating his own food requests at whim and per his appetite. And it was like witnessing firsthand a miracle. I had begun seeing him grab food from the fridge or take second helpings on his own. He now pounded sodas like a middle school boy. And he licked the sugar off his fingers from the delicious malasada treats (local Polynesian donuts) he liked. Each sign had been one more arrow indicating we were heading out of that dark valley. Now I realized the valley was behind us. What I wanted to do was jump for joy and do the victory dance. I matched his smile instead and grabbed him that desirable bowl of goodness. And then he got up himself and added a nice tall glass of bone-strengthening milk. He usually drank two glasses these days with his meals. Not his required one. Milk does a body good.

Got milk?

Brother maintained those gains and continued them through another summer. A summer that involved sports and friends and most amazingly *healthy and uninhibited eating*. At his one year mark since the day of his diagnosis, he had actually grown two inches in height and upgraded two shoe sizes. By 2015, he added an astonishing six more inches in height and it seems likely the starvation was arrested in time to deter any long-term impact to his growth potential. This only happened because of the quick re-feeding regimen that occurred and the strict adherence to the treatment model! He outgrew his mother and was happy about it! The physical gains have been incredible, but the mental progress is what indicates the healing is hopefully here to stay. He has come to a place of not just accepting the growth process, but celebrating it! His goals involve "getting as tall as he can", "getting stronger," and becoming a "professional athlete," and his method is to eat when hungry and listen to his body cues. He wears a proud smile when he opens jars his mother cannot and loves easily showing me up in the strength department! He miraculously passed eighth grade and began high school with a truly new start and new mindset. His freshman year report cards were evidence of intellectual healing, astoundingly demonstrated by a cumulative GPA of 4.0! He sees an accurate image in the mirror and is no longer triggered by his reflection. He exudes confidence and positive self-regard. Now I am sure, like all of us, he will have insecure moments and thoughts of self-doubt. Nonetheless, he has courageously and successfully eradicated the *with*. He is now Brother. Period. Not Brother *with* anorexia. He genuinely likes himself and seems to accept himself for who he is. Another family *food for talk* dinner time, the question posed was "Name one thing you like about yourself." His answer "Because I am me." Amen, Son.

> ***Tip #25:*** *Notice the five senses and what they reveal. Be open to what this information brings you, and acknowledge what is happening "here and now." Don't be tempted to distort reality when the information is disheartening. Put in the hard work up front, with swift and immediate action to reverse this horrifying illness. Your life and your normal will be put on hold and altered drastically, but a return to an even better normal can be at the end of that journey.*

Don't hide your scars;
wear them as proof that God heals.

— Jarrid Wilson

CHAPTER 26

THE VALLEY OF THE SHADOW OF DEATH—IS BEHIND US

I have three purposes in writing down our family's journey and victory over anorexia.

First, I want to point to the heavens and give glory where glory is due. I believe in the God of the Bible, and this belief goes deeper than *because the Bible says so.* I witnessed the hand of God heal my son. *He* healed through Angel Ingrid and her wisdom and breadth of knowledge in the world of eating disorders and the complexities of this devastating killer. *He* healed through her referral to Roger's Memorial. *He* healed through Dr. Ulland at Rogers who taught "energy in before energy out." *He* healed through a team of experts who stood together for life and nourishment. *He* healed through Angel Kirsten, who shed tears and cared for my son daily with love in action and responded to death threats with calm and unconditional acceptance. *He* healed through Angel Angie who sat with my boy through every snack and countless lunches for an entire school year. *He* healed through a 504 plan and school staff who came together and said they would do what it takes to support this child. *He* healed through a college quarterback who cared enough to hit "Send." *He* healed through a nutritionist who did blind weigh-ins. *He* healed through a mother's love. *He* healed through the child himself.

You see, the God who created us and knows us intimately and finds us unconditionally lovable is bigger and stronger than anorexia. In fact, the lies of anorexia are diabolically opposed to His message of love and acceptance.

> *John 10:10*
>
> *The thief comes only to steal and kill and destroy. I came that they may have life and have it abundantly.*
>
> *Psalm 139:13-16*
>
> *For you formed my inward parts; you knitted me together in my mother's womb. I praise you, for I am fearfully and wonderfully made. Wonderful are your works; my soul knows it very well. My frame was not hidden from you, when I was being made in*

> *secret, intricately woven in the depths of the earth. Your eyes saw my unformed substance; in your book were written, every one of them, the days that were formed for me, when as yet there was none of them.*
>
> *Proverbs 4:20-22*
>
> *My son, be attentive to my words; incline your ear to my sayings. Let them not escape from your sight; keep them within your heart. For they are life to those who find them, and healing to all their flesh.*

In Brother's journey, as in the journey of mankind, the path was prepared before the demons and angels entered the scene. For Brother's health, the divine preparation began in the form of a request in the Spring of 2013. Before he knew what he needed in the near future, he requested we move. This middle school child began asking his mom to move to another valley. A move that made no sense! His request was to start the next school year in a district far from where we resided at the time, in a neighborhood I did not think I could afford. It made zero logistical sense in terms of commute and work and the life we were setting up. I look back in awe. That summer while my son was an ocean away, slowly starving, and I was oblivious to the danger lurking, I proceeded to seek housing in the vicinity of his preferred school. My rationale: to listen to my son and his needs and to start him off in a school district where he would have some youth group friends. And during this time, a new friend at church, Angel Kirsten, generously offered to watch my boys before and after school. This kind of offer is not something that happens to single moms frequently!

God knew. And had plans in place to carry His child through this storm. God provided a home in a very competitive rental market at a price I could afford. I moved on faith alone. When I went to retrieve my very ill son, I brought him back to a new home—one he had never set foot in. A home divinely located within a few drivable miles of his entire treatment team. A home that was in the only school district I have ever heard of as providing such amazing care and support, which enabled his healing. A home literally smack dab between the homes of Angel Ingrid and Angel Kirsten, the very people God would use to be His hands and feet and mouth. God was active and alive in all these moving parts. It amazes me to think that the God of the universe loves my son this much. He loves us all. I hope you consider His love in your life.

Secondly, I have to honor my son. I have to honor his struggle and his pain and find the meaning behind it. His condition had the tragic effect of compromising his mind—and I am not sure what the years will continue to bring in terms of recall and recognition of all these pages conveyed. Some things he has forgotten, repressed, or not realized about his symptoms. In part, I write this book because if one did not watch this journey up close and just met my son today, they wouldn't believe it ever happened. He is now the epitome of health and positive self-regard. I want him to know what he has overcome. I want him to recognize his resilience, his inner strength, and his recovery. The bravery and courage he demonstrated to face his fears and push through them every time food was placed in front of him despite a terrorist screaming in his head is incredible! His persistence through unimaginable internal pain speaks to his character and drive. This was indeed a family battle, yet Brother was the true victor. The winning warrior. His strength to overcome was the determination of the outcome. He was the one who, moment by moment, hour by hour, meal by meal, had to filter the chaos, force down each bite, and drown out the voice of the enemy who sought his demise. He trusted the helping hand until that beautiful moment in time when he could trust his own mind again. I have never before witnessed such tenacity and valor! My hope is for Brother never to forget his capacity for healing and never lose sight of the joy in coming out of the dark valley (*Psalm 23*).

My third purpose in penning this narrative is the very real desperation I felt as a mother watching her child slip away in the grip of Terrorist Joey, and empathizing with and wanting very much to prevent this for other helpless victims and their families. I don't want any other child or adult to suffer needlessly through this. And I know many currently are. I want to provide hope, hope for healing. Hope for a life without eating disorders. I want to silence the barrage of self-denigrating thoughts. I want to strengthen the message of value and inherent worth and personal power. I hope to eradicate Terrorist Joeys everywhere. I want to share what worked in our case and pray that it empowers and aids someone in pain somewhere.

> *2 Corinthians 1:3-4*
>
> *Blessed be the God and Father of our Lord Jesus Christ, the Father of mercies and God of all comfort, who comforts us in all our affliction, so that we may be able to comfort those who are in any affliction, with the comfort with which we ourselves are comforted by God.*

Your life has great significance, Son. Live it fully.

Love,

Mom

> ***Tip #26:*** *Life is precious—and we are put on this planet for a purpose. Know your purpose and be assured that you can survive the dark valley and so can your child—and a celebration of health and healing can be accomplished.*

What is done in love is done well.

— Vincent Van Gogh

A FINAL NOTE

HEALING YOUR CHILD'S HIJACKED MIND

As a parent, we are not required to be sideline observers to anorexia's course. I acknowledge that we have limited power, but claiming the power and authority and privilege we do have...we can be our children's most important advocate. After reading Brother's story, what actions are you going to take? Has eating been negotiable or non-negotiable in your home? Has Terrorist Joey invited himself into your four walls and sat down at your dining room table with his legs wrapped around the post legs, refusing to budge? Some parents may believe themselves helpless to kick him out.

I challenge you to distinguish your child's voice from that of his or her terrorist. I challenge you to do what is in your child's best interest and directly opposed to the desires of the Eating Disorder. I encourage you to choose *food* for your child. Children *get* to eat.

It is a gift. A gift of life. Do not align with or enable the illness. Do what you can to rid your child of his or her hijacker. Use this book as a reference and a reminder of hope in this battle. Research the Maudsley Approach: Family Based Treatment, and consider its potential value in your child's treatment.

In the exercise lines below, jot down the top ten actions you will commit to taking immediately as a result of reading this book:

> Ex: Contact the Eating Disorder Association of America (1-800-931-2237; info@NationalEatingDisorders.org) and find local treatment specialists

1. ______________________________
2. ______________________________
3. ______________________________
4. ______________________________
5. ______________________________
6. ______________________________
7. ______________________________
8. ______________________________
9. ______________________________
10. ______________________________

In this book, you learned about the dangers of an underfed, malnourished mind. You learned about the eating disorders: anorexia and bulimia. You read of strategies to regain the cockpit of a child's hijacked mind. And you equipped yourself with tools to gain some momentum. I wish you and your child health, safety, and a full recovery. May you once again also hear the blessed phrase, "Mom, what's for dinner?"

Jessica Goering, LMHC, NCC

We acquire the strength we have overcome.

— Ralph Waldo Emerson

EPILOGUE:

BROTHER IN HIS OWN WORDS

Experiencing this devastating illness firsthand truly taught me how valuable life really is. However, as I look back on the past and those fateful days when the illness began to blossom and consume my mind, I still struggle to remember everything I went through. Whether I have repressed the memories too deeply or malnourishment from that time has hampered my memory, I cannot seem to connect all of the dots. However, with every fiber of my being, I can confirm that my mind was hijacked and that it was not truly my real self making those life-threatening decisions.

Throughout the entire process, I thought I was doing what was "right" or "healthy." That thought process could not have been further from the truth. I cannot stress enough how much I needed a parent or someone outside of me to ensure recovery when I could not choose what was true health for myself. I needed a rock in my life during those unsteady times. As I have read through my mother's book, I have been hit by a flood of memories and emotions. I am forever grateful to my mother and truly do not know where or if I would be here today without her intervention.

Reversing Your Child's Eating Disorder: Healing a Hijacked Mind to Overcome Anorexia is an outstanding resource for any caregivers out there who are currently facing the terrible disease of anorexia nervosa. It is almost impossible to describe the mental torture and internal storm I was experiencing, which is why anorexia can be so difficult to figure out how to treat. However, I know I was in desperate need of swift and enforced treatment. As Angela Guarda, director of the Eating Disorders Program at Johns Hopkins University, puts it: "The longer you have anorexia, the more anorexia creates physiological changes in the body and the brain that then create a self-sustaining cycle." The key here is to transform how struggling victims are handling situations mentally. Teaching them a healthy mental approach will allow them to see themselves more accurately, thus leading to physical progress. Additionally, for their mental side to see itself properly, it absolutely needs nutrition and to be re-fed first and foremost. However, sufferers will never choose food for themselves. I know I would not and could not have. They need someone to lead them through this internal darkness so they can emerge with a renewed sense of self and a new mindset about the world. In conclusion, caretakers have an absolutely vital role to play in healing their children from this horrid affliction. I can 100 percent attest to the fact that the tips and strategies throughout this book were critical for my recovery, and I want my story to help those who are struggling like I was.

My mother wrote down our story hoping it would help me remember and heal, and it truly has. Her decision to make our story public was also contingent on my approval. After reading the book, my exact words were "I highly encourage it, and I hope it can be used to help others."

I am sure the reader is curious about how I am doing now. I am very happy to share that I have been in remission without relapse since overcoming this ordeal. However, I still struggle at times with a tendency to put too much focus on food, and I am especially vigilant about healthy foods. Yet I have learned how to take care of myself and my health. As of this date, I have demonstrated my remarkable recovery by graduating with the rigorous and highly regarded International Baccalaureate Diploma (IBDP) from my high school. At graduation, I was bestowed the honors of valedictorian, summa cum laude, and academic honors while being an active athlete throughout my high school career. My personal highlight was being selected as a varsity football captain my senior year. Now I am attending college and am embracing the future. None of this could have happened if it were not for the life-saving enforcement and recovery instilled by my mother, with the help of so many amazing helpers in my life. I remember the "Angels" and all they did for me, and I am truly grateful for their unconditional support throughout that dreadful journey. Accepting my story helps me to understand what dangers and pitfalls to avoid and how to differentiate true health from the lies of a distorted perception of "health." Likewise, I truly hope this book can be a powerful tool in fighting the dangerous grip of anorexia nervosa in your child's life.

Yours truly,
"Brother"

Even in the darkest phase, be it thick or thin, always
someone marches brave here beneath my skin.

— K.D. Lang

TEN CLUES AN EATING DISORDER HAS HIJACKED YOUR CHILD'S BRAIN

1. **Eating Patterns Change**
    - Subtle or sudden avoidance of certain food items, especially sweets and calorie laden foods
    - Binge eating, periods of high food volume
2. **Distancing Socially**
    - Becomes isolated from others
    - Avoids interactions with family and friends
3. **Hobbies Avoided**
    - Interests, clubs, sports, activities that used to be requested/enjoyed no longer are

- Lack of enjoyment is noticeable to attentive observer

4. **Image Fixation**
    - Obsession with scales, measuring tapes, body checking in mirrors
    - Body comparison with other people and self-degrading talk

5. **Justification of Privacy**
    - Secretive behaviors centered around food and eating
    - Requesting or demanding to eat alone/unwarranted time spent in bathroom

6. **Anxiety and Moodiness**
    - High levels of anxiety, especially fear of being fat
    - Irritability, lower frustration tolerance

7. **Calorie Counting**
    - Increased interest in food content
    - Tracking of calories or fat grams

8. **Keeping Body Hidden**
    - Changes in physique/appearance, especially weight loss
    - Attempts to hide such changes

9. Excessive Movement

- Calorie burning of any kind (exercise, pacing, obsessive physical drive)
- Unnecessary motor activity

10. Dramatic Shift in Personality

- Unexplainable change of how child "is in the world"
- Interactions with others of different nature/intensity

Although the world is full of suffering,
it is full also of the overcoming of it.

— Helen Keller

TEN WAYS TO HELP YOUR CHILD OVERCOME THE EATING DISORDER

1. **Overcome Denial**
    - Observe with your five senses what is happening with your child
    - Face the reality of what is happening; fight the urge to deny these changes
2. **Very Quickly Seek Medical and Professional Help**
    - Take this seriously and seek treatment ASAP
    - Research experts in the field and consider Maudsley Intervention
3. **Eating needs to be Non-Negotiable**
    - Take back parental authority in the eating department

- Your child has a brain disorder that will prevent him or her from personally choosing food; you as the parent need to choose it for your child!

4. Reach out for Support

- You can't do this effectively alone
- Build a support team to ensure your child is not able to engage in destructive eating behaviors without accountability

5. Challenge Irrational Thoughts

- Child's brain is deprived of nutrition necessary to make rational thoughts and choices
- Need to stay rational as the parent and reframe these thoughts through therapy

6. Obsessive/Compulsive Urges Need to be Stifled not Reinforced

- As the anxiety spills out in strange, odd behaviors, prevent expression of them as much as possible
- Be a barrier to these behaviors—do not reinforce them

7. Monitor Eating Continuously until Weight is Managed

- Never give your child a chance to engage in destructive eating urges
- Be firm, consistent, and expect compliance

8. Externalize the Illness

- Your child is not the eating disorder; your child has an eating disorder and needs your help to rid his or her mind of these intrusive and irrational fears—verbalize this separation
- Distinguish the child you love from the behaviors that are hard to deal with

9. Empathize with Your Child

- Your child is being required to face his or her biggest fear (fat) through eating...numerous times daily!
- Be empathetic and kind and compassionate; tough love implemented consistently is a powerful change agent

10. Decrease Control over Food Choices as Your Child Increases Healthy Eating Patterns

- Gradually shift control over food back to your child as he or she regains an ability to make healthy food decisions
- Baby steps are required here, but you have to give your child opportunities to succeed and regain trust in this area

You have control over your thoughts,
and unless you take control of them,
they will take control of you.

— David DeNotaris

TERRORIZING THOUGHTS

FOR PARENTS TO CHALLENGE AND REFRAME

Distorted Thinking	***Rational Thinking***
"I must be skinnier to be okay."	"You are okay just the way you are."
"Food makes me fat."	"Food keeps you alive."
"I will feel better and be happier if I don't eat."	"Your brain chemicals trigger depression and anxiety when not fed."
"I'm fat."	"We don't talk about superficial body descriptions in this family."
"I must be perfect."	"Perfection is impossible. It is a setup. Mistakes help us learn."

"No one likes me."	"I like you, ____ likes you, and ____likes you. What does the evidence say?"
"I will never be good enough."	"Your worth is not determined by what you do or what you see in the mirror. You are good enough for who you are."
"Everyone thinks I am fat."	"You cannot read minds."
"You hate me."	"I decide my feelings. I love you."
"If I eat that, I'll get fat."	"Some fat is essential to stay alive. Food has other purposes in our body."
"I don't want to grow up."	"Growing up is hard, but becoming an adult gives you freedom and power."
"I can control those horrible feelings when I don't eat."	"When the brain doesn't have fuel, the horrible feelings increase."
"I am worthless."	"You are a valuable and significant person."
"I am a failure."	"The evidence is you are successful at _____ and _____ and _____."
"I hate food."	"I know eating is hard for you right now. You don't have to like it. You do have to eat."

"I caused this."	"Anorexia is a brain disorder. Not a chosen experience. You are not responsible."
"I will never get to eat how I want!"	"You used to have full control over eating until anorexia invaded. You will get full control back when anorexia leaves."
"I will never get out of treatment!"	"Treatment is temporary. You will get your life back and this will end."

Nothing in life is to be feared;
it is only to be understood.

— Marie Curie

RECOMMENDED READING

Brave Girl Eating: A Family's Struggle with Anorexia by Harriet Brown

Eating Disorders in Children and Adolescents: A Clinical Handbook edited by Daniel Le Grange and James Lock

Eating in the Light of the Moon: How Women Can Transform Their Relationship with Food Through Myths, Metaphors, and Storytelling by Dr. Anita A Johnston

Eating with your Anorexic: How my Child Recovered Through Family-Based Treatment and Yours Can Too by Laura Collins

Family Therapy for Adolescent Eating and Weight Disorders: New Applications edited by Katherine L Loeb, Daniel Le Grange, and James Lock

Help Your Teenager Beat An Eating Disorder by James Lock MD, PhD and Daniel Le Grange, PhD

Life Without Ed: How One Woman Declared Independence from Her Eating Disorder and How You Can Too by Jenni Schaefer

My Kid is Back: Empowering Parents to Beat Anorexia Nervosa by June Alexander and Professor Daniel Le Grange

Rationale and Principle Interventions in Family-Based Treatment (Fbt) for Adolescent Anorexia Nervosa by James E. Lock and Daniel Le Grange

Skinny Boy: A Young Man's Battle and Triumph Over Anorexia by Gary A. Grahl

The Oxford Handbook of Child and Adolescent Eating Disorders: Developmental Perspectives by James Lock

Treating Bulimia in Adolescents: A Family Based Approach by Daniel Le Grange and James Lock

Treatment Manual for Anorexia Nervosa, Second Edition: A Family-Based Approach by James Lock MD PhD, Daniel Le Grange PhD and Gerald Russell MD

RECOMMENDED RESOURCES

Emotes Action Figures

Food for Talk: created by Julienne Smith

Maudsley Parents
www.MaudsleyParents.org

National Eating Disorder Association
www.nationaleatingdisorders.org

What lies behind us and what lies before us are
tiny matters compared to what lies within us.

— Ralph Waldo Emerson

REFERENCES

(1) http://www.apa.org/helpcenter/eating.aspx

(2) Insel, Thomas. (February 24, 2012). Director's Blog, Spotlight on Eating Disorders. http://www.nimh.nih.gov/about/director/2012/spotlight-on-eating-disorders.shtml

(3) http://www.anad.org/get-information/about-eating-disorders/eating-disorders-statistics/

(4) Myers, David. *Exploring Psychology*. 9th ed. New York: Worth Publishers, 2012.

(5) http://www.ncbi.nlm.nih.gov/pmc/articles/PMC1414759/

(6) http://www.eatingdisorderexpert.co.uk/lanugoandeatingdisorders.html

(7) http://glossary.feast-ed.org/5-psychology-and-therapies/ego-syntonic

(8) http://www.mirasol.net/blog/outsmart-eating-disorder-brain-fuel-pt-1/

(9) http://www.maudsleyparents.org/maudsleymisconceptions.html

(10) http://www.maudsleyparents.org/whatismaudsley.html

(11) http://train2treat4ed.com/fbt-for-anorexia-nervosa/

(12) http://abcnews.go.com/Health/Wellness/eating-disorders-prevelant-kids-twelve/story?id=12238077

(13) http://www.mirror-mirror.org/teens.htm#sthash.HOTCqtuF.dpuf

(14) Johnson, Rick. *That's My Son: How Moms Can Influence Boys to Become Men of Character*. Revell, Grand Rapids Michigan, 2005

(15) https://www.sciencenews.org/article/anorexic-brain

(16) http://www.eatingdisorderhope.com/treatment-for-eating-disorders/types-of-treatments/family-therapy

(17) http://www.cancer.org/cancer/cancerbasics/questions-people-ask-about-cancer

(18) http://ghr.nlm.nih.gov/glossary=generegulation

(19) http://www.aipono.com/teen-program-founder-message

(20) Peck, M. Scott, M.D. *People of The Lie: The Hope for Healing Human Evil.* A Touchstone Book: Simon & Schuster, New York, 1983.

[21] https://www.theguardian.com/society/2016/mar/29/anorexia-you-dont-just-grow-out-of-it

Pain insists upon being attended to.
God whispers to us in our pleasures,
speaks in our consciences,
but shouts in our pains.
It is his megaphone to rouse a deaf world.

— C.S. Lewis

ABOUT THE AUTHOR

JESSICA GOERING is an author, professional keynote speaker, psychology adjunct instructor, national board certified counselor, and licensed mental health counselor. She has a Bachelor of Science in Psychology degree from Liberty University, a Master of Arts in Counseling Psychology from Bowie State/European Division, and has studied the field of psychology and human behavior for eighteen years. Jessica has taught psychology courses at the college level for ten years—including Introduction to Psychology—and Developmental Psychology. She has worked with children and adolescents as a school-based mental health counselor, has provided therapy services to the community as an advanced clinician and has specialized training and extensive experience working with military populations. She is a parenting and family advocate trained in Bowenian Family Coaching and has been a workshop presenter for the European Branch of the American Counseling Association conference.

Jessica has held her favorite title, *Mother*, for eighteen years and has applied her professional insight to the rearing of her own children and helping them maneuver the challenges of being raised in a single parent home. She knows firsthand how important personal resiliency is and how to encourage and foster its course in lives around her. She has spent time volunteering in programs such as Celebrate Recovery, for those who struggle with addictions; New Beginnings Crisis Pregnancy Center, for those who find themselves with an unexpected pregnancy and need emotional support; as well as the Wounded Warrior Program, for physically and psychologically wounded service members. Additionally, she finds great meaning in mentoring and encouraging other parents in their roles as heads of households.

Today, Jessica lives on Oahu, Hawaii, with her youngest son who is a high school freshman while Brother is a college freshman studying on the mainland. She enjoys sharing life with her church Ohana (family) and admiring the creative power and majesty of the Most High God. She spends her time actively building community and loves investing in the physical growth, emotional health, and spiritual development of both her children.

Jessica is passionate about her work in the mental health field and helping families heal from the trauma of anorexia. She is optimistic that this book will find its way into the hands of those who need to find hope and healing for their child's hijacked mind.

Contact Jessica at:
(808) 798-9979
www.JessicaGoering.com
www.ReversingYourChildsEatingDisorder.com
Jessica@ReversingYourChildsEatingDisorder.com